No matter how much
I needed this book when I was young,
it wasn't meant for me.
I needed to tell my stories here and now instead.

~ SNA ~

For all of you who work hard to "get up" every day,
and to Lisa who has taught me more about
getting up than anyone (besides myself).

~ DN ~

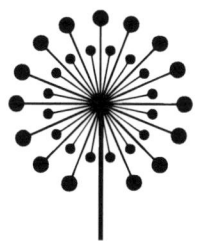

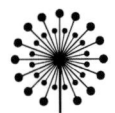

The Get Up Book

Text copyright ©2021 Sharon Neiss

No part of this publication may be reproduced, stored in a retrieval system or transmitted, in any form or by any means, without the prior written consent of the publisher or a licence from the Canadian Copyright Licensing Agency (Access Copyright).

All quotes and references have been cited, otherwise all original content written by Sharon Neiss Arbess and David Newton

Printed in Canada/Globally

Project development, management & strategy
by Borden Communications + Design Inc.

To order books, book programs, order accessories or for any other inquiries,

> This book is not intended as professional medical advice, diagnosis, or treatment. Always seek the advice of your physician or other qualified healthcare provider.

WELCOME!

When Sharon arrived in to my office for a consultation, she wasn't looking to write another book ... she was looking for a way to support you, your mental health, and your emotional intelligence. At the time, I had also started my new venture, The Akira Concept, with David, who had over three decades of working in fitness and wellness and teaches movement like no one I had ever known - not in my personal life nor through my business.

When Sharon expressed that she wanted to write stories and help youth, I knew that I had to connect them. Most of us love to learn in "chunks" or "tidbits" and so Sharon, David, and I decided to pair short stories that would make you nod your head and feel seen and heard with simple and functional movements to stack into your daily life. It's a book that you now hold in your hands ... and it's something that we all wish we had at your age.

I believe that everyone is their own best expert - that means you are your best expert and know what's best for you. However, when we have conversations with other good humans (who have open minds and open hearts), we can learn so much. In the spirit of this, we decided to include advice from many others who care about you too - this isn't a book with one voice. What I didn't realize until reading through all of the submissions from our "mentors" was that so many of us "older adults" wish they had been weirder, bolder, stronger, and louder themselves ... less concerned about what others thought. Perhaps this is the biggest lesson for me that I have received from being part of this book with Sharon and David ... the understanding that hindsight for most on the other side of youth wish they had been more of themselves at your age. I certainly know I would have!

As you read Sharon's short stories and learn and practice David's rituals, remember that the challenge or struggle might just have the answer for you to thrive. Hold that thought. It is an important truth. Once you learn it, your world will change. So many of our personal issues (and world issues) come from us abandoning ourselves. Stick with yourself, you're worth it.

Good for you for making the commitment to Get Up. Don't lose touch with your first step ... which you have already taken. There are a lot of people that poured their hearts and souls into this book and are cheering you on!

Lisa

Lisa Borden
Producer of Get Up, Unconventional Idealist, Innovator, Instigator and Initiator.

It's all about the why, what, you, and me.

WHY I needed to write this book.

WHAT makes me qualified?

WHY should YOU listen to ME?

I am fascinated by the teenage years. They are overflowing with an abundance of change. The body growing at rapid speed, along with demanding academics and social life.

While everyone goes through this time in their life, I believe they need, at some level, mental health support - be it professional, from a parent, a friend, or from me. I am a writer, storyteller, and "resiliency mentor" who "gets it". From what I saw, experienced, and went through myself, I am able (and delighted) to share my stories that are hopefully meaningful, relevant, and full of lessons - things that I wish I knew when I was your age. Most of the stories are true and others are a product of my imagination. As for movement, moving well makes you feel better, and the exercises that David has paired with my stories will help you feel great in your body, mind, and soul.

I assure you that you are not alone.

If this book helps you get through your day a little bit easier, I will feel as though I've done my job.

Welcome to my vault!
Enjoy the ride - I sure am!

Sharon

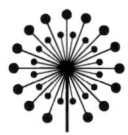

HOW TO USE THIS BOOK
It's time to GET UP

Whoa - what's all this?
Just a little preview to what's in store in the pages to follow.

Each chapter in Get Up has four main parts.

The story part: Each story that I've written is "based" on some sort of truth. Most of them have been twisted around for privacy and creative reasons. Any writer will tell you that the best part of the job is playing the puppeteer. Regardless to where my imagination took me, the bottom line is that these stories are lessons that I wish I knew when I was a teen.

You may relate to them. Or not.
Some stories may also bother you. Or not.

Read them anyway.
Read them to a friend.
A parent.
The person who cuts your hair.
Ask them what they think too.

Read them again in a month or so.
You may have a different view, as your life changes.
And it will.

The movement part: Written by David Newton. First there is The Ritual (why do you need to do this exercise) and then there's The Practice (the exercise itself).

Some are strenuous while others are more sedate and relaxing. When you get to this part of the chapter and you want to practice it, make sure your body and the place you choose to exercise is ready. Empty your bladder, make sure you've eaten in the last two hours. Wear comfy clothes. Doing squats in platform shoes may not be the best idea, neither is swinging your arms when there are breakables around.

The Mentor part: We called on some pretty amazing people to share a few words of wisdom that they wished they could have told their teen self. Sound familiar? As successful as they are, they too have gone through some pretty tough times - and learned from it.

The space to write part: After reading and doing, your head might be swarming with good stuff that you've got to write down, right? Scribble. Sketch. Pour your thoughts down on that paper. This book is yours and yours to keep. Some stories and advice can stir up a lot of feelings that need to be expressed and be placed somewhere that can be reflected on at a later time. We wrote what we think, now it's your turn.

But really... We're not looking over your shoulder, so you can read it any way you like, but in order for it to make sense, we suggest treating each chapter as a whole. Start from the title and make your way through. But feel free to jump around each chapter.

And, for any terms that might be unfamiliar to you (or that we made up), you can find our definitions in the glossary at the back of the book.

It's time to Get Up and have fun!

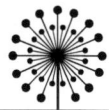

TABLE OF CONTENTS

How to GET UP in 30 Chapters

CHAPTER 1 1

Take Care of Your Body ... It's Your Home for the Rest of Your Life
What to do today, to keep you standing tall tomorrow.
PROUD SHOULDERS

CHAPTER 2 9

Strength and Struggle
Someone's Strength is another person's struggle.
THE HELP-ME PUSH-UP

CHAPTER 3 17

Sitting Isn't the New Smoking
How to counteract negative aspects of sitting, because we all sit.
THE BUTT LIFT

CHAPTER 4 25

Self-Imaging
How you see yourself is what matters.
THE SUPERHIGHWAY

CHAPTER 5 33

Why "Later" Won't Work
If you put off stuff to do tomorrow, tomorrow will be today.
GET A MOVE ON

CHAPTER 6 41

Why Are You Following Me?
Repeated characters that keep popping up in your life.
ENERGETIC CORD CUTTING

CHAPTER 7 49
When Will It Be My Turn?
Waiting for things you want to happen.
THE TUMMY BUSTER

CHAPTER 8 57
Short-Term Pain for Long-Term Gain
It will only hurt for a short time and the results will be worth it.
THREE BRAIN MEDITATION

CHAPTER 9 65
Lost and Found
You never know when someone will rise to the occasion.
3D LIVING

CHAPTER 10 73
Make Your Bed
Watch the domino effect happen. Magically.
WINDSHIELD WIPERS

CHAPTER 11 81
Mood Swinging
Own your mood and act accordingly.
GET YOUR "FEEL GOOD" FIX

CHAPTER 12 89
It May Look Perfect But It Ain't
*It looks like the grass is greener,
but it may be fake grass and other things too.*
THE SLALOM

CHAPTER 13 97
One Door Closes and Another Opens
When a door is locked, it may be for a reason.
STANDING CAT/COW

CHAPTER 14 105
Great-Full
Gratitude practice, a healthy habit that we all need to do. Especially now.
FEELING GOOD ABOUT ME

CHAPTER 15 113
Salad Master
There is more than one way to eat your greens!
THE LUNGE MATRIX

CHAPTER 16 121
It's All Perspective
Change your way of thinking, which will in turn change your view.
GAZE SHIFTING

CHAPTER 17 129
Just Keep Cleaning ... Just Keep Cleaning
Housekeeping for your soul.
THE HELICOPTER

CHAPTER 18 137
Letting Go
As you make a change, you never know what you will reinvent.
OFF-ROAD-SPEED-PLAY

CHAPTER 19 145
Whoa
Stop that galloping horse. Stop for just a moment and think.
START BY STOPPING

CHAPTER 20 153
The Magic of Failure
It's humiliating and painful, but you need it in your life.
I CAN'T DO THIS!

CHAPTER 21 161
Find Your People. Know Your People.
Choose your friends wisely.
THE BIG SQUEEZE

CHAPTER 22 169
FOMO VS JOMO
Are you missing out for the right reasons?
TRUST YOUR GUT

CHAPTER 23 177

Get (Para) Sympathetic
Controlling your nervous system.
IS YOUR WINDOW OPEN

CHAPTER 24 185

Getting Rooted
*Fast foot facts and why you should care
about where and how you stand.*
FEET ON THE GROUND

CHAPTER 25 193

Change the Scenery
Choose wisely on what you want to look at.
AROUND THE WORLD

CHAPTER 26 201

Centered Strength
It's amazing what can throw you off balance.
GUT PUNCH

CHAPTER 27 209

Motivation and Discipline
They seem the same, but they're so different.
THE MOTIVATOR

CHAPTER 28 217

21 Days to Form a Habit
Before you know it, it will be like second nature. It just takes a little practice.
21 DAY PUSH-UP CHALLENGE

CHAPTER 29 225

From BFF to SFF
The changing of a friendship.
THE SIDE BEND

CHAPTER 30 233

Catch Your Breath.
When it all becomes too much, take the time to just breathe
HIIT

Take Care of Your Body ...
It's Your Home for
The Rest of Your Life

*What to do today,
to keep you standing
tall tomorrow.*

You can become strong, powerful and beautiful.

VENUS WILLIAMS

Take Care of Your Body ...
It's Your Home for The Rest of Your Life

What to do today, to keep you standing tall tomorrow.

It's hard to imagine what you will look like when you're old. When I was very young, I used to scrunch up my face and think about how I would look when I grew older. Obviously that didn't happen.

I bet you don't even want to think about it either. You have other fish to fry. School commitments with a laundry list of tests and papers to write. Presentations too. Who's doing what with whom on your screen. No doubt that the teen years are for the here and now.

How can you think about what you will look like in 20, 30 or even 40 years from now?

The answer to that question came right in front of my daughter and I one morning en route to school.

There he was. A man slightly older than her father. He was walking, hunched over. I mean really hunched over. Like he was bending over to pick up something, but he wasn't. He was walking in that painful looking physical state to the subway.

"How does he get measured for his height at the doctor?" My daughter bluntly asked me.

"He doesn't." I replied.

"_____" She answered with her eyebrows raised.

Kyphosis is the condition, which is commonly known as "Hunchback" and it affects between 20-40 percent of adults. The culprit? Sedentary lifestyles and lack of exercise. The amazing thing is you can prevent this from happening; however, it's not a quick fix.

Partaking in weight bearing exercise by using your body weight and/or barbells are incredible for your bone and muscular health. Exercises like these don't have to be excruciatingly difficult and they shouldn't cause pain. They just have to be hard enough that they make you want to stop when you get to the 8th rep.

Aside from the sports, active extra curricular activities, and the daily walk to school, you should set aside some strength training time as well. Approximately 10-15 minutes a day.

If you start now when you're young, and make this a healthy habit you will be way ahead of the game. And you will be standing super straight, too!

THE MORAL OF THE STORY:

It's your body, and you need to take care of it.

Weight bearing exercise helps all daily activities, including the sport that you play. It will also help you stand up straight and also be able to lift your grandchildren!

Ritual: Proud Shoulders

Your posture introduces you before you do.

Did you know that people judge you by the way you carry your shoulders?
Do you realize that you probably judge others the same way?

Your "Kinesiosphere" is the auric energy that you are enveloped in and it is the energy that you share with others. It is how you show off your mood and emotions. Proud posture and shoulders give off confident, strong, and happy energy and stooped shoulders display poor health, sadness, and a lack of confidence.

Understand that your mind's connection to your body is very real ... and very powerful!

You naturally have a much easier time keeping your shoulders strong when you are young because you aren't yet carrying the long term "weight of the world" on your shoulders. As you get older, if you don't take care of your body, the added responsibility of day to day stress can eventually, over time, take its toll on your body and posture.

The most significant thing about poor posture is that it is completely avoidable and it can be fixed. By keeping your back, shoulders, and core muscles strong and your shoulders and chest stretched open, you will, in turn avoid a number of problems like chronic back pain, fatigue, headaches, and poor self-esteem.

With just a little extra daily effort you can retrain yourself to avoid poor posture and its negative side effects. With just a little effort you can stand tall today, into adulthood, and beyond.

Practice: Proud Shoulders

THE REVERSE FLY

How to do Proud Shoulders:

Stand in a comfortable position with a slight bend in your knees and your feet about the same width as your shoulders.

Bend forward from the hips until your back is almost parallel to the floor.

Let your arms hang down beneath the shoulders.

With your elbows slightly bent raise your arms out and away from the sides of your body until they are at the same height as the shoulders.

Pinch your shoulders together like you are trying to juice an orange.

Slowly lower the arms back down to the starting position.

The reverse fly is an exercise that we can do to target the postural muscles of the back and shoulders.

Don't do this:

Don't collapse the spine.

Don't hunch the shoulders forward.

Don't hold your breath during the exercise.

Do this:

Keep the natural position of the spine throughout the exercise.

Keep your elbows and your knees soft at all times.

Keep the movement of the forward bend and arms smooth and controlled at all times.

THE BOTTOM LINE:

Beautiful and proud posture is the result of having a strong back and shoulders.

Mentor Memos

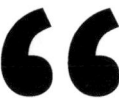

Do not adjust yourself
to fit into society;
be yourself and let
society adjust.

Marci Warhaft

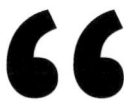

It doesn't matter what other people
think of you and you do not need
to change or try to be like anyone else.
Dare to be different from the
big group, if that is who you are.
There is no inherent value in sameness.
Be yourself and be proud of who that is.

David W. Eisen

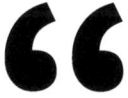

Don't get too caught up in
what people think of you.
Who the $&@# cares?
Just be you.

Gordie Arbess

Connect The Thoughts!
Jot down notes and self-reminders here.

Strength and Struggle

Someone's strength is another person's struggle.

**Where there is
no struggle
there is no strength.**

OPRAH WINFREY

Strength and Struggle

Someone's strength is another person's struggle.

It was that time of year again. Parent and teacher's Interviews. When it was time to meet Mrs. R., my son's math teacher, I cringed. This meeting was obviously not for my evaluation, but I was still nervous. Math was not my strongest attribute when I was young and as I walked down the school corridors to meet her, I said, "Happy Times!" to myself with great sarcasm.

Nothing got by Mrs. R. Strict with plenty of sass. That was her claim to fame. Some thought her blunt personality was funny. Others, not so much.

When it was our turn to meet, she got right to the task at hand. I casually made a joke about how I struggled with math as a kid. She looked me straight in the eyes and said, "I can't choose paint colours. We are redesigning my bedroom right now and every time we work on it, my body clenches up like a spider hiding from it's predator."

My jaw dropped open.

"Excuse me?" I asked, feeling shocked out of my mind. I added "How can decorating your room be stressful? You're just picking new furniture and choosing a nice new paint colour. Maybe an area rug, too". I looked at Mrs. R. with curiosity. How could she not get excited over this? I was getting excited. And it's not my bedroom!

Mrs. R. smiled at me and said "We all have our struggles. Mine is with decorating. Yours is with numbers. It's just how it is."

"Do you have a decorating tutor? Because I had a math tutor," I said.

"You can say that." She giggled.

"Decorating anything is out of my comfort zone. I'm not used to it - I find it very stressful."

"I agree, but with this stuff." I pointed to the math textbook.

Before we knew it, our time was up. "What about my son?"

She lifted her finger and said "Right! He's doing fine. He finds math exciting!"

I left the classroom smiling.

THE MORAL OF THE STORY:

View your strengths as your gifts and view your struggles as a challenge. Working through your struggles will teach you and others that it's OK to be outside of your comfort zone and try hard things.

Ritual: The Help-Me Push-Up

Training with someone else can have so many benefits ... try it and you will quickly see! It is also a great way to challenge your body to go outside your own comfort zone ... the overall gains can be huge.

Did you know that working out with a friend can be more fun? Did you know that it can also challenge you to be more accountable and make you push yourself harder?

A friend can be a great motivation to get a really good workout. If you have committed to a friend, you will be more likely to show up and give it your best! It's almost impossible to say you're skipping your workout when you have someone waiting for you and counting on you.

Your workout buddy can push you to become stronger and faster. They can also provide you with valuable guidance and feedback - remember, you can't see yourself when you are working out the same way someone else can! It will also give you a chance to support your friend.

The Partner Assisted Push-Up is the perfect way to learn to work (and workout) with another through struggles with supportive strength. How great will it feel to have the assistance of someone to help you get through the more challenging parts?

A workout buddy will help you stay safe and encourage you to work your body's full range of movement.

Some things are just better when done together!

Practice: The Help-Me Push-Up

PARTNER ASSISTED PUSH-UPS

How to do The Help-Me Push-Up:

There is no special equipment needed, just a friend and a towel.

Have the person you are helping lie down on the floor, face down, and have them place their hands on the floor slightly wider than their shoulders.

Have them step their feet out behind them into a high plank position and remind them to keep their body in one giant straight line.

Straddle their hips and loop your towel under their chest.

Encourage them to lower down towards the floor slowly and assist them back up, using the towel.

Switch places and let your workout buddy do the same thing for you.

Don't do this:

Don't hold your breath.

Don't collapse your spine.

Do this:

Let your partner assist you through the tough parts.

Exhale when you're pushing yourself away from the floor.

Keep your spine in a neutral position.

Work from your knees instead of your toes when you get tired.

THE BOTTOM LINE:

A good friend will not let you wimp out in your workouts! They can help you to become stronger faster and you can do the same for them!

Mentor Memos

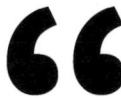

Care more. Everything and everyone matters.

Linda Kessler Shapiro

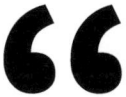

You are capable of giving and deserving of receiving transcendent love.

Megan Khosroshahi

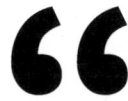

Friendships are give and take:
Their upkeep and nurturing is a shared role.
Be generous and give space to let those
you love and trust, offer that same
support back — and graciously accept.
We can gain valuable insights and
lessons from all of our relationships —
whether they are brief, ebb and flow,
last a lifetime, or otherwise.

Wendy Chong

Connect The Thoughts!
Jot down notes and self-reminders here.

Sitting Isn't The New Smoking

How to counteract negative aspects of sitting, because we all sit.

**It's not that I'm so smart,
it's just that
I stay with problems longer.**

ALBERT EINSTEIN

Sitting Isn't The New Smoking

How to counteract the negative aspects of sitting, because we all sit.

"Have you got Ass-Power?"

"Excuse me?" I asked with my eyebrows raised.

"You know. Ass-Power." She said again. Clearly. As if I didn't hear her.

Oh, I heard her.

"Ass-Power is the ability to sit down and work. For hours."

I was still staring at her. Thinking.

I assumed that my dinner guest had these powers because she is a physician and in order to get to do what she does everyday - you need to sit your ass down and study for a very long time.

This type of focus and attention needs to be done when you want something. Badly.

Such as figuring out algebra, reading Macbeth, conjugating French verbs or memorizing your lines to a play.

You are sitting for a reason. To absorb information so you can get to the next step (or grade, or level). And then you get to do this, which leads to that and then you can do that all day long, which is your lifelong dream.

In order to add a little health-kick to this regime, how about this:

Get up from sitting every two hours and walk around. Get outside for a leisurely stroll, or even a run and get your heart rate up. It will help you absorb the information and keep you focused.

But don't forget about sitting to just relax. And doing nothing. Ok, nothing and screen time. Yes, there is time for that, too. With a physical break of course. When night falls and it's time to catch your zzzzs, all electronic devices should be placed out of your sight (at least 30 minutes before bed*).

Especially before bed!

Direct quote from my 16-year-old daughter: "You know, when I put my phone away and read before bed, I sleep much better."

So sit. Absorb. And, get up and move, too. The results will be so worth it. For "That".

*National Sleep Foundation

THE MORAL OF THE STORY:

Blocking off time to study will test your discipline and motivation to get to a goal. Practicing hours of study will prepare you for challenging projects which will require your focused concentration.

Ritual: The Butt Lift

If you learn how to squat properly you will boost your Ass-Power!

Did you know that your butt gives you the power to walk and run?

When you sit your butt muscles don't work. If you sit for long periods of time, your butt goes to sleep. Squats are a very simple and easy way to wake up and strengthen these muscles. They are not only good for toning, but butt power also directly supports your knees, spine and your overall health.

Squats help strengthen many other lower body muscles and are known to build and enhance balance and movement. They challenge your core to work hard and even more so when done with a barbell or dumbbells.

They can be done anywhere anytime because all you really need is your own body weight. You can do many different kinds of squats and each one will affect the butt and leg muscles in a different way. It is important to learn how to squat correctly so that you don't hurt your back, knees, hips, or ankles.

Practice: The Butt Lift

THE SQUAT

How to do The Butt Lift:

Stand in a comfortable position with your feet slightly wider than your hips. You can change the position of your feet to change the way your muscles work.

Using your body weight to do the squats, raise your arms to shoulder height to help with balance. **OR** place a barbell on the muscles at the base of your neck for additional weight. **OR** hold a set of dumbbells in your hands next to your hips as you squat for additional weight.

Place your body weight equally on both feet.

Slowly sit down (and back) as if you are sitting into a chair.

Stop when your hips are slightly higher than your knees.

Use your butt to slowly raise your body back up to the starting position.

Don't do this:
Don't move too quickly.
Don't hunch or round your back.

Do this:
Make sure your hips, knees, and ankles all move when you are squatting.
Keep your feet firmly planted on the floor.
Keep your neck in a comfortable position.
Make sure you keep your core muscles engaged
to support your lower back and hips.

THE BOTTOM LINE:
Power and shape come to those who squat!

Mentor Memos

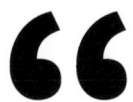

"There is no learning without pain. And that's the step most of us miss. To truly understand something, it's got to hurt.

Leslie Josel

"Your path is your own and you can blaze your own trail.

Christopher Wong

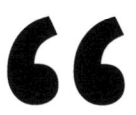

"Took me a while but my advice is nothing.

You must go through all the bumps and bruises yourself to learn and grow from your own journey.

So no advice.
Go through it.
Learn from it.

Sandy Kruse

Connect The Thoughts!
Jot down notes and self-reminders here.

Self-Imaging

*How you see yourself
is what matters.*

**You are responsible for
what you say and do.
You are not responsible for whether
or not people freak out about it.**

UNKNOWN

Self-Imaging

How you see yourself is what matters.

At my first job, I was approached by my manager to lead a new project.

The first few weeks of meetings and brainstorming sessions went well. But as the months went on, I began to twirl my hair between my fingers and think. A few more meetings went by and I no longer twirled my hair but began to rub my temples. It became clear to me that there was a problem.

The project team was not being productive and I had to make a change. People weren't doing their jobs and other colleagues noticed a growing rift in the team.

In an attempt to improve the situation, I moved people's positions around and gave them a list of what needed to be done. Not only did I stir the pot, but I dumped it out, and created a whole new dish!

The question you might be thinking here is how did everyone feel?

Not so good.

How did I feel?

Not so good either.

The process of taking control and changing people's positions around was uncomfortable and emotionally painful as I have never done that sort of transaction before.

Change is hard on people. It creates an uneasiness that may lead to a negative reaction.

I began to see myself as negative and harsh.

"But you are in charge of how you see yourself," someone wise said to me.

"But I'm such a bitch!" I exclaimed back. I felt guilty. Shameful. Harsh.

"But things weren't working the way it was before. You had to make this change."

My friend was right. My job was to be in charge of this project and if that meant I had to take a stand and move things around, that's what I had to do. Respectfully, of course.

With some self-reflection, I began to see myself as a leader who was making a positive and productive change. Eventually, my colleagues adjusted to their new roles, and I and everyone else was pleased with the end results.

I was not a bitch.

THE MORAL OF THE STORY:

Whether you are the leader of a project team or decide to wear your favourite green T-shirt for the entire month of September, it is YOU who decides which reactions are welcome into your subconscious that will in turn create the self-image of yourself.

Ritual: The Superhighway

If you learn how to breathe well, you will be able to do so much more in life! Breath is like a Superhighway between your mind, body, and soul.

Did you know that breathing is the only self-regulating system in your body that you can control?

Your breath is the most powerful and readily available tool that you possess when it comes to connecting with yourself on all levels. Breath is critical in our day-to-day health, well-being, and longevity. It is also one of the most misunderstood and confusing natural body functions.

If you practice breathing when you are in a relaxed position, then when you are in a more stressful situation you will be able to manage and cope better. If you develop your own healthy breathing habits now, and understand why you are doing them, you will find that they will serve you for life and you will be able to stand up straighter ... strong and tall.

Your breath is also an indicator of your mood and your mood is an indicator of your breath. This means that if you change how you breathe, you can change your mood. It also means that when your mood changes, so does your breath.

You can use your breath to calm yourself, to increase your energy, support exercise, reduce anxiety, and aid in recovery and healing.

Remember: It's not about the destination, it's about the journey on your Superhighway. Just imagine, when you practice belly breathing it has the power to help you do everything in life better.

Practice: The Superhighway

BEDTIME BELLY BREATHING

How to do The Superhighway

Lie down face up in a comfortable position.

Place and keep your hands on your belly.

Inhale. Feel your hands rise. **they will when you breathe from your belly!*

Exhale. Feel your hands fall. **they will when you breathe from your belly!*

Continue for twelve breaths.

Feel the calm.

Don't do this:

Don't be judgmental.

Don't change the way you breathe ... just breathe the way you do!

Do this:

Keep your breathing relaxed.

Pay attention to the rising and falling of your hands.

THE BOTTOM LINE:

Breath is everything. Connect with it.

Mentor Memos

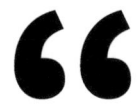

> You will find your time.
> For context, my teenage self was quite shy,
> unsure of who he was,
> wanting to be someone else
> and generally angry with the world.
> I'd tell him not to worry about the
> coke bottle glasses, the lack of muscles,
> the lack of success with the ladies
> and the clumsiness.
> I'd tell him, you'll find your place
> in the world and your tribe
> where you are appreciated.
> I'd tell him to appreciate his uniqueness
> and to listen to his intuition and
> be "unashamedly you".
> I'd also reassure him that it will be a
> constant journey of rediscovering himself
> and that he is a beautiful human being – that
> he doesn't need anybody else to tell him that!

Nicholas Ferguson

Connect The Thoughts!
Jot down notes and self-reminders here.

Why "Later" Won't Work

*If you put off
stuff to do tomorrow,
tomorrow will be today.*

Do it now because it's not going away.

LESLIE JOSEL

Why "Later" Won't Work

If you put off stuff to do tomorrow, tomorrow will be today.

Dinner is over and there is a pile of dishes in the sink.

You have two options.

1. Do the dishes = Do it now.

2. Leave the dishes = Do it later.

Number one is hard and let's face it: you don't want to do it. Who does? Especially if the sink is filled with so much stuff! I mean, where do you start? You can't even see the bottom of the sink because it's loaded with dishes, food and guck. It's a total mess.

Number two is super easy and way awesomer! If there is such a word. All you have to do is look at the mess, smile and take off! Yee ha! You can even say "See ya LATER!"

But here is the kicker. What about LATER? When is later?

The feeling you have, let's call it *meh* when you first see the dishes will be the exact same feeling later. Meh. I can guarantee that you will not feel elated or filled with joy and anticipation when you decide to do the dishes LATER.

It's almost like taking your medicine to get rid of strep throat.

You take it now and it tastes awful.

You take it later and it still tastes awful.

Bottom line: It has to get done (the medicine, the dishes, whatever you need to do) to get the result you want (a clean sink, no more strep throat or whatever you want done).

The only way to do the dirty dishes deed is to make NOW more exciting because you can control the environment you work in.

Put on some "dishes music".

Strike up a conversation with your "dryer".

Listen to a podcast.

And the feeling afterwards? Pure joy! Why? Because you accomplished a job that was a challenge.

THE MORAL OF THE STORY:

Some jobs are boring, hard and not exciting. It's all part of life. Chores, like the dishes, must get done. Who else is going to do it? We all have to do our part.

As mundane as chores may be, studies show that tasks like dishes, teach teamwork, responsibility, respect and a strong work ethic.

Ritual: Get A Move On

We have to take responsibility for our own health and well-being and this involves self-discipline and a strong sense of dedication to moving our bodies every day.

Did you know that power or "fitness" walking is an amazing way to exercise and that it doesn't require any special equipment or athletic ability?

One of the main pillars of character building is taking responsibility for your actions and understanding that there are always consequences for those actions that can be both good and bad. Sometimes it is easier to grasp "responsibility" when we flip it around and focus on the outcome or the "consequences" ... for example, a sink full of dirty dishes. The dishes have nothing else to do but sit there and be dirty. They will win every time! If you don't do them they don't get done! It all boils down to you being accountable to yourself first, and then having an understanding about how your actions affect those around you. It's about understanding that we all have duties and that we can either approach them with, "I have to" or "I get to". Our approach or mindset can make a huge difference when something needs getting done like dishes or the day to day responsibility of keeping ourselves fit and healthy.

Yes, you have a responsibility to your body and to keeping it fit and healthy! The consequences are that it has a positive effect on you mentally, emotionally, and physically. One of the easiest ways to build fitness and health is to power walk. Getting yourself moving not only helps tone muscles and build strong bones, but it strengthens your immune system, your heart and lungs, enhances your mood, as well as boosts brain function and power.

You can keep your walks challenging and interesting by changing the speed, by adding intervals, and by walking on uneven surfaces like trails, stairs, and hills. Power walking is a solid workout for your hips, back, and legs and at the end of your workout you will probably be more fatigued than you might think. It's a good idea to start slowly and build your workouts over time. Ultimately, your walks should be challenging, enjoyable and, of course, kind to your body.

Practice: Get A Move On

POWER WALKING

How to Power Walk:

Keep your head and chin in a normal upright position.

Keep your shoulders proud (upright and chest open) ... always stay strong in your posture.

Your elbows should be bent to 90 degrees and they should swing close to your body.

Gently pull your belly button in toward your spine so that your core muscles engage and support your movement.

Relax your hips and think about moving your body forward.

Take short steps and make sure that your heel is not pounding into the ground when you step forward.

Don't do this:

Don't let your shoulders slouch forward.

Don't flail your arms.

Don't make your steps too big.

Do this:

Always stay connected to the surface you are walking on and your surroundings.

Be creative with the routes you take your walks on.

Make sure you wear comfortable shoes and clothing that you can move freely in.

Get off the road and into nature!

THE BOTTOM LINE:
A good solid power walk will leave you feeling joyful and will lead to being motivated to walk again and again!

Mentor Memos

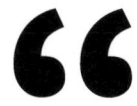

> Everything that you learn is worth it,
> even if you are not sure how,
> when, and where it will be useful.

Leanne Matlow

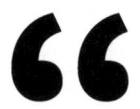

> Don't eat cereal for breakfast
> it makes you hungry and tired —
> instead get a good blender and
> have fruit and vegetable smoothies
> and you will have much more energy!

Melanie Levcovich

> Don't be afraid to
> shine your light.

Betsy McLeod

Connect The Thoughts!
Jot down notes and self-reminders here.

Why Are You Following Me?

Repeated characters that keep popping up in your life.

**Good relationships feel good.
They feel right.
They don't hurt.**

MICHELLE OBAMA

Why Are You Following Me?

Repeated characters that keep popping up in your life.

Whether you are on the playground, standing near your locker, or in front of your screen, there will always be that person who drives you crazy.

And as you grow up, you may notice that the same type of person repeatedly shows up in your life.

For instance, when you were in the second grade, there was that girl who pulled your hair when she wanted your juice box. Now that you are in the 7th grade, there's this guy who likes to slap you on the back (a little too hard) as a friendly greeting.

These personalities will follow you at each stage of your life. They could be helpful and mentor-like or cruel and narcissistic.

If it's the latter two, how do you respond to this? How do you catch it from repeatedly happening?

I remember my friend Laura bought a pair of concert tickets and she asked one of her friends to go with her six months in advance.

A week before the concert, the friend had to cancel. The reason was not an act of God (a tragedy in the family or illness). She unfortunately refused to pay for or sell her ticket which forced Laura to scramble at the last minute to sell it.

And she didn't feel good about it.

Ten years later, Laura's phone rang and it was a friend from university who was in a panic.

She was two hours away, attending a wedding.

"Laura! You know the dress I packed?"

"Yeah......" Laura asked.

"It sucks! I hate it!" She screamed.

Laura sat there in silence, not knowing what to say.

"Can you bring me your velvet green one? With the bow at the back?"

Laura got in her car, and delivered the dress.

She didn't feel good about it, again.

Several more instances occurred, with different characters and different scenarios, but with the same outcome and she felt like she was being treated like a chump.

Why doesn't Laura learn from her past experiences and reject those that mistreat her?

She hasn't learned how to properly react to this unacceptable behaviour.

Yet.

THE MORAL OF THE STORY:

Take a look at your choice of friends. Do they control your every move? Do they convince you to do things that you're uncomfortable doing?

These repeated instances create an uncomfortable feeling that is preventing you from taking control of your life. Catch the pattern of mistreatment and put a stop to it. It will prevent any future occurrences and the ability to refuse what you don't want to do. Choose friends that will not treat you like a chump, but a champion.

Ritual: Energetic Cord Cutting

Not only are we physical beings, but we also have a strong spiritual and energetic side as well.

Did you know that you share this energy with your friends, families, neighbours, and co-workers every day?

Energetic bonds or connections happen naturally between you and the people in your life and in order for them to be positive and healthy, these bonds need to be full of trust, love, and self respect. Sometimes you form these connections to people who have selfish, disrespectful, and harmful intentions toward you. This bad energy can make you feel sick, nervous, and often leads to anxiety, depression, and poor self esteem.

A really good way to manage bad relationships and the way they make you feel is to check in with yourself first and to understand what is at the root of your own frustrations and discontent. Another positive way to deal with difficult people is to talk to them. Communication is a healthy way to honour and respect your own feelings and it is also a great way to understand, process, and deal with the way the other person is feeling.

Energetic cord cutting is a positive way to remove bad energies between you and others so that the effect of these negative friendships doesn't hang over you or impact the way you live your life. Feelings like anger, anxiety, and sadness can be recognized, removed, and replaced by other more positive feelings, thereby making room in your life for supportive and positive friendships. Cord cutting will not make the other person disappear but the practice can give you the confidence to be happy and positive with yourself even when you have to share space with them.

Letting unhealthy relationships go is a process and if you practice cutting these negative cords with dedication and consistency they can help you remove these bad energies from your life. Cord cutting is a simple and healthy way to help you release the negative energy bonds that you form with others. It is a great way to build and enhance self-respect and also a powerful way to foster mental and emotional health and wellness.

Practice: Energetic Cord Cutting

CORD CUTTING

How to do Cord Cutting:

Find a quiet place where you can sit, stand, or lie down.

Close your eyes and begin focusing on your breathing.

Think about the person that you wish to cut cords with.

See the negative energetic cords that you have with this person and their connection to you.

Envision yourself cutting these cords so that they are no longer connected to you.

You can use your hand in a chopping motion to remove the cords.

Repeat this process as often as needed until you feel they are gone.

Finish the process by replacing the cords with feelings of gratitude and appreciation for all of the good people you have in your life.

Don't do this:

Don't despair, the process takes time and patience.

Don't worry about the person with whom you are cutting negative cords.

Don't be harsh or critical about yourself.

Do this:

Believe in your ability to change and remove something that is negatively affecting you.

Give yourself permission to live your life free from the relationships that do not honour you.

Believe that you deserve to be happy!

THE BOTTOM LINE:

You can find peace, happiness, and forgiveness when you learn how to cut negative energy cords.

Mentor Memos

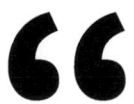

> Don't be afraid to be weird.
>
> *Ryan Storm*

> Beware of "Compare and Contrast". As soon as we do this, as girls and as women, we put ourselves at an immediate disadvantage. Embrace your smarts. Your body. Your tastes. Your preferences. Your opinions. Your fashion statements. Your playlists. Your interests. Learn to trust your own passions and instincts and surround yourself with people who love you and truly want what is best for YOU.
>
> *Debbie Berlin*

Connect The Thoughts!
Jot down notes and self-reminders here.

When Will It Be My Turn?

Waiting for things you want to happen.

**Patience is bitter,
but the fruit is sweet.**

ARISTOTLE

When Will it Be My Turn?

Waiting for things you want to happen.

12-year-old Stacey was in history class, trying to pay attention to what was being taught. It was hard to concentrate due to the whispers and giggles from her classmates.

It was Friday afternoon.

A party was taking place that night.

The school bell rang.

A bunch of kids jumped up, squealed and made a mad dash to the classroom door. Stacey watched how they were all beaming with excitement as they grabbed their stuff from their lockers and raced to the staircase that led them outside.

Stacey remained at her desk. She continued to watch the camaraderie until all was quiet.

"Aren't you going to leave, Stacey? It's Friday afternoon! Go - have a great weekend!" Chirped her teacher, Mrs. G.

"What's the point? I'm not going to that party." Stacey quietly said.

"I see…you know, you can't dance at every wedding."

Stacey squinted her eyes at Mrs. G. out of confusion.

"What I mean is, it's okay to not be at every party."

Stacey turned her head towards the window. Her eyes began to fill with tears, which she quickly wiped away with her hands.

"Some parties won't be worthwhile for you."

Stacey turned to Mrs. G. and looked at her as if she had three heads.

Mrs. G. continued, "These kids that are having this party. Do you usually hang out with them?"

"No," Stacey quietly said.

"Then why do you think you would like to go to a party with them?"

Stacey looked up and began to think.

Mrs. G. leaned in and whispered. "You haven't gone to THE party… yet."

"But when will I? When will it be my turn?" Stacey asked.

"It will happen. You'll see."

THE MORAL OF THE STORY:

Respect the timing for certain things to happen in your life.

Whatever your "want" is, you may have to wait for it and trust that it will eventually happen when the time is right for YOU.

Ritual: The Tummy Buster

The main purpose of your core is to provide foundational support and power to your whole body.

Did you know that your core is responsible for good posture?

When you think about it ... when you really think about it, did you really want to go to that party? A party with a bunch of kids that you don't even hang out with. Maybe they're the "in crowd", but are they *"your"* in crowd? Take a moment to understand the root of your feelings ... are your wants misguided? Much like the roots of a tree, there is great value in knowing and understanding the roots of your thoughts.

Your greatest happiness and accomplishments will always happen when your thoughts and actions have deep roots. You must trust these inner thoughts and believe that they will lead you to feel happy. This is certainly one of the most important lessons that you will learn in life! Being successful is an amazing experience but remember that it is always the byproduct of all of the little steps (and big ones) that you experience in your day to day journey.

Recognizing your own self-worth is also important and a deep understanding of the self takes patience, thought, and time. Sometimes when you really think something out, (like the party that Stacey wasn't invited to) you realize that it was something that probably wasn't really that good for you and it wouldn't have made you happy. Remember that each day will be full of choices ... embrace them and be grateful that you have deep roots.

Your body's root is your core and when it is strong it makes everyday tasks like carrying your backpack, daily chores, and running, much easier. The supine bicycle crunch is an amazing way to build core strength and is a lot more challenging than sit ups because it adds rotation to your workout. The crunch also builds power in your back, shoulders, and legs. If you are patient, disciplined, and diligent you can build awesome core power.

Practice: The Tummy Buster

SUPINE BICYCLE CRUNCH

How to do The Tummy Buster:

Start by lying flat on your back on the floor.

Place your hands behind your head and raise your feet off the floor (keep your knees bent to 90 degrees and stack them directly above your hips).

Raise your shoulders off the floor.

This is your starting position.

Gently twist your spine and bring your right knee and left elbow together.

At the same time extend your left leg out.

Return to your starting position.

Gently twist your spine and bring your left knee and right elbow together.

At the same time extend your right leg out.

Return to your starting position.

Repeat the exercise both ways until you feel your core muscles work.

Don't do this:

Don't strain your neck by pulling on the back of your head.

Don't do this exercise if you feel pain in your lower back.

Don't forget to breathe.

Do this:

Always stay in control of the speed of your movement.

Exhale when your elbow and knee come together.

Inhale when you move back to the starting position.

Pay close attention to how your lower back feels and modify the exercise if you feel pain or tension.

THE BOTTOM LINE:
Strong core = strong posture and movement.

Mentor Memos

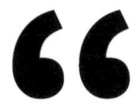

> Always respect yourself and know your worth.
> There will be situations that will test and try.
> You and your self-esteem may take a hit -
> do not allow life's hiccups to define you.
> Be patient and kind with yourself as you would
> with anyone you love, respect and trust.

Debra Basch

> Follow sparkly people—
> humans who stand out
> in their ability
> to listen to their own heart.
> Being close to them
> will allow your own
> thrum to sound clear.

Hope Paterson

Connect The Thoughts!
Jot down notes and self-reminders here.

Short-Term Pain for Long-Term Gain

*It will only hurt
for a short time and
the results will be worth it.*

**There are
no gains
without pains.**

BENJAMIN FRANKLIN

Short-Term Pain For Long-Term Gain

It will only hurt for a short time and the results will be worth it.

Dear A,

I can't believe I'm here. It's only been 8 freakin' days. I have 21 more days and 11 hours to go in this hippy-dippy freaky flower child drug rehab dungeon. Get me outta here.

I really need a hit. Literally like now. I am aching for it. Just one more time.

LATER

OMG - I just heard there's some Molly on my floor. I just need to give them my wool sweater. Don't need it anyways.

LATER

I am waiting. Waiting for it. A bunch of us are by the library. Pacing. My leg can't stop twitching. My heart keeps beating so loudly, I am sure everyone can hear it.

I keep playing with my sweater. Spinning it around. Making a knot with it. I stare down at it. I stop and think. My grandmother gave me this sweater. What am I doing? Why am I here? What am I getting again?

I run outta there so fast, clutching my wool sweater. I run to my room. And cry. And cry some more, holding my wool sweater. Why would I trade something so beautiful, so wonderful for one more lousy hit?

AFTER

My urge to get high is still here, but I know I can't trade in my sweater that my grandmother gave me - that's crazy. Why do I need to get high? I have 21 more days and 9 hours to find out.

THE MORAL OF THE STORY:

Although what you are going through may feel uncomfortable and even painful, this feeling will eventually stop and you will experience an awakening. A growth and change from where you started.

Ritual: The Three Brain Meditation

Persistence and patience will give you the skills to overcome your struggles and obstacles.

Did you know that the process of learning and understanding something new involves our brain being uncomfortable and confused?

In life, learning or adapting to something new always involves the process of training your brain to understand. Your understanding will result in some kind of change and this may involve periods of confusion, discomfort, adaptation, and finally, improvement. Something that was initially very hard and thought to be impossible gradually becomes easier to understand and something you can handle with less difficulty and struggle.

It has been scientifically proven that you have more than one brain in your body. In fact you actually have three! Who knew? The brain that you are probably most familiar with is your head brain. It is your thinking brain and where you form reasonable and sensible thoughts based on accurate and logical information. For example, figuring out a math problem.

Your second brain is located in your heart centre. It is your emotional brain and where you feel emotions such as love, hate, fear, happiness, and pleasure. A great example of this is the reaction you have to someone you love. And finally your third brain is located in your gut. It is your intuitive brain and where you form instinctive thoughts. Have you ever said to someone, "I feel it in my gut?"

Learning about and making change to addictive behaviour involves all three brains working together like an orchestra. They need to be constantly communicating, influencing each other, and learning and adapting to new coping skills. The three brain meditation gives you the opportunity to understand each brain and its sensations as well as how each brain influences and relates to the other two.

Practice: Three Brain Meditation

THE VISUALIZATION

How to do The Visualization:

Choose a comfortable position, close your eyes, and focus on connecting to your breath. Open yourself up to learning about yourself during this meditation.

Think about connecting to your logical brain that is located in your head. Slow your breathing down and let this in turn slow your thoughts down as well. Spend as much time here as needed to create a connection to your breath and stillness.

When you are ready, start thinking about connecting to your emotional brain that is located in your heart centre. Slow your breathing down and let it radiate from your heart. Let your breath move between your head and your heart and feel the connection of these two brains.

Once again, return to your breath and think about connecting it to your intuitive brain that is located in your gut centre. Visualize a strong and balanced connection between your gut, heart, and head centres.

Let your connection to your breathing move you among the three brains in any way the meditation takes you.

Your breath is a very powerful tool in this meditation so when you find your mind wandering just slowly return it back to breath.

Don't do this:

Don't be critical, judgmental, or force your breathing and connection to your three brains. Don't expect anything specific, let the meditation take you where it will. Don't forget to move yourself through all three brain centres.

Do this:

Believe in the possibility of a strong and harmonious connection to all three brains. Make sure you are comfortable during your meditation. It is okay to sit, stand, or lie down. Let your breath be your guide.

THE BOTTOM LINE:

Challenge yourself to embrace and learn something new every day! Appreciate the power that your breath holds!

Mentor Memos

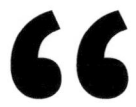

> Put yourself out there
> and take more risks.
> Don't be too concerned about
> what your peers would think, which
> may result in playing it "safe".
> Setbacks are an
> important part of success.
> No one achieves anything
> worthwhile without trying,
> failing, getting back up,
> and trying again.
>
> *Martin Perelmuter*

> You are a super connector
> and that is a super power
> because connections are powerful,
> they build love, community, and
> those are building blocks for resiliency.
>
> *Peter Neal*

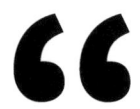

Connect The Thoughts!
Jot down notes and self-reminders here.

Lost and Found

*You never know
when someone will rise
to the occasion.*

**Be kind whenever possible.
It is always possible.**

DALAI LAMA

Lost and Found

You never know when someone will rise to the occasion.

While visiting my sister in Colorado, I stayed in a hotel, which had a really inviting and cozy lobby. There were these great big pillowy couches that faced enormous windows that showcased Colorado's beautiful mountains. This spot quickly became my go-to place to hang out.

One morning, as I was tip-tapping on my laptop on one of the cushy couches, my bracelet was bothering me. It kept clanging on my keyboard and making a scratching noise. I decided to take it off and so I slipped it in my purse and went on with my day.

The next day, in my hotel room, I reached for my wrist, and my bracelet wasn't there. My heart dropped to the floor. I spilled out my purse, moved chairs, stripped my bed, and got on all fours and searched every inch of my room. Nothing.

I usually wear this bracelet when I travel and am away from my children. I like to play with the gold blocks that spell their names. It's as if they are with me at all times.

I darted back to the lobby and took off all of the cushions from the couch where I usually sat. A hotel employee came by and asked me what I was doing. I explained the situation and was told a notice would be sent out to all hotel employees.

This bracelet was insured. I knew exactly where I got it and could replace it, but it didn't matter. I wanted this bracelet, the original one that I lost. As silly as it seemed, even though it was just a "thing" this was my favourite piece of jewelry that meant a lot to me and I had an emotional attachment to it. It was part of me.

"It's gone." I complained to my sister.

"Wait. Have some trust, someone may find it and return it to you."

I wanted to believe her, but I also accepted the fact that it may be gone.

After a day out on the town, we both returned to the hotel to check with the concierge to see if anything had come up. And there, in the corner of my eye, on the hotel reception desk was my bracelet shimmering in a plastic bag.

I found the person who returned the bracelet and thanked him profusely. He just stood there and smiled and said "You're welcome." This whole scenario didn't seem to faze him. Perhaps in this man's eyes, this behaviour was his norm. To follow the simple rule: You find something that isn't yours? Return it. No matter what it is.

My sister and I hugged each other and jumped up and down like we won the lottery. And I truly felt like I did. In humankind.

THE MORAL OF THE STORY:

Appreciate the kindness that people can bring everyday. The more kindness you experience, the more it can be contagious and you will have more hope.

If you find something that isn't yours, find the owner.
They will be grateful.

Take good care of your stuff!

Ritual: 3D Living

You spend a good part of your day getting up and getting down (on and off the floor, into and out of chairs, car seats, couches, and more) and you need to make sure that your body stays happy and healthy so that you can continue to do this comfortably and easily.

Did you know that you need both upper and lower body strength when getting up and down off the floor?

Rule #1: You must love and express kindness toward yourself before you can offer real love and kindness to those around you ... now say this again and understand that these words are meant for your ears to hear most. Rule #2: You must also show compassion and cultivate positive thought toward yourself before you can truly offer these beautiful gifts to others ... now say this again and embrace it, really embrace.

It may seem odd at first but you can learn these behaviours ... anyone can learn these behaviours. Practising these thoughts, expressions, and actions can lead to positive changes in the way you think and behave, and this will ultimately lead to so many positive shifts in your body, mind, and soul. "Loving kindness" toward yourself and others can make you feel really good! It can reduce stress and anxiety, boost your mood, self-esteem, self-worth, and self-confidence, and ultimately have a positive and healing affect on both your physical and emotional pain. Being in this mindset will enable you to reciprocate, like the hotel employee who found Sharon's bracelet.

Movements that take you from a standing position to getting down and up off the floor are a big part of the way your body is supposed to naturally move. Think about getting into and out of a bathtub, sitting on the ground, reaching for something on a high shelf in your closet, or reaching for something under a low table or under your bed These movements all rely on overall body strength, flexibility, and both upper and lower body mobility to make them happen. The All Terrain is the perfect exercise to wake up your whole body and to keep it strong no matter the position you're in!

Practice: 3D Living

THE ALL-TERRAIN

How to do The All-Terrain:

Stand in an upright position.

Raise your hands over your head and reach for the sky.

Squat down and place your hands flat on the floor shoulder width apart.

Step your feet out behind you and move into a high plank.

Bend your elbows and lower your body to the floor.

Push yourself back up into your high plank.

Walk your feet back up to your hands.

Return to a standing upright starting position.

Raise your hands back up to the sky.

This is one complete All-Terrain.

Do as many as you feel comfortable doing.

Don't do this:

Don't collapse your spine in high plank.

Don't move too quickly.

Don't forget to breathe.

Do this:

Do the push-up from your knees to make it easier.

Engage your core, hold your spine in a strong position during the push-up.

Try to establish smooth and fluid flow through the whole sequence.

THE BOTTOM LINE:
Practicing loving kindness can lead to better self-understanding and empathy toward others.

Mentor Memos

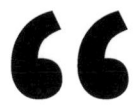

> I'll borrow from Don Miguel Ruiz - Be impeccable with your word!
>
> *Navaz Habib*

> Life sometimes gets in the way of your dreams. But, if you look at your life as part of the journey to attain your dreams, you won't feel as much pressure to try and figure it all out right now.
>
> *Stacey Jackson*

> Love is where the magic lies and gives us wings to fly.
>
> *Krystyna Roberts*

> Every minute you worry about how your friends will react is 60 seconds you could be doing something far more valuable.
>
> *Naomi Strasser*

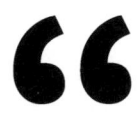

Connect The Thoughts!
Jot down notes and self-reminders here.

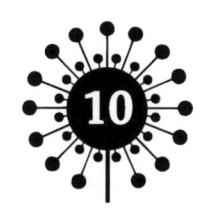

Make Your Bed

*Watch the
Domino Effect happen.
Magically.*

**If you want to
change the world,
start off by
making your bed.**

WILLIAM H. McRAVEN

Make Your Bed

Watch the Domino Effect happen. Magically.

The other day I stood in the doorway of my son's room.

"Make your bed." I said.

"Nph." That was his version of "No."

To make a point, I set my timer from my phone right near his elbow. He was doing homework at the time and he stopped what he was doing to watch me.

I made his bed in one minute and 36 seconds.

His room looked "Done." "Finished." "Ready."

"Ta daahhh! See?" I proudly said.

You have so many things on your plate.

Making your bed is a starting point that will get your engine running to tackle the upcoming responsibilities ahead.

Once you begin with a made bed, try taking your clothes off of the floor and put them away. Notice how your head feels clearer? Ready to address what needs to be done? Cleaning up the rest of your room also helps create a "Domino Effect" of good habits and wise choices for the rest of the day.

We urge you to try it. Once the sheets are tucked in, your comforter is laid out and you place the pillows in their places, a tidal wave of euphoric energy sweeps into your body. You can't help but smile and feel proud.

Don't be surprised if passers-by take notice and offer a compliment or two. Who doesn't like that?

In less than two minutes, a chore can be crossed off of your list and you can have that great "I did it" feeling. Quick, painless and totally doable. If only chemistry could be just as easy.

I know what you're thinking - whatever happened to my son and his bed? Did he begin to make it? Put away his clothes?

He just moved into his student apartment in university and not only did he put together his furniture, but he made his bed.

THE MORAL OF THE STORY:

Just start.

The simple act of making your bed causes an immediate sense of accomplishment, which will lead to a Domino Effect of smart habits for the rest of your life.

Ritual: Windshield Wipers

Your hips are second only to the shoulders when it comes to body flexibility and joint motion.

Did you know that your hips are the most important part of your body when it comes to moving through your everyday activities?

The "Domino Effect" is a chain reaction where one thing or task triggers similar events ... good things lead to good things. This effect can be applied to your behaviour, like when you take on one thing like making your bed, and how this has the potential to lead to other such things like picking up your clothes, etc. ... you know what I mean. This cascade of events can lead to feelings of accomplishment which can in turn make you feel better about yourself.

The routines and habits that make up your daily life are all interconnected. Focusing on, and sticking to just one can lead to other positive changes like the increased focus when you're writing essays and studying for exams, even though this wasn't your original intention. Following through leads to good intentions, good intentions lead to action, and before you know it you will be surprised at how easy and beneficial it is to get your daily chores done.

There are 17 different muscles that give power and flexibility to your hips and if just one of these muscles is not doing its job then your hips are compromised ... the "Domino Effect". The strength, flexibility, and general health of your hips cannot be taken for granted! Not only are they the primary joints when it comes to your body being able to move but they also have a direct relationship to the power and flexibility of your your knees and back.

Your hips support your weight when you sit, stand, walk, and run. In order for your hips to be healthy and do their job, they need to be flexible. Supine CHAMPs is a really easy and efficient way to make sure that all of the muscles that support your hips stay elastic and healthy. The "Windshield Wiper" is an active moving stretch that ensures that your hips stay mobile and strong forever!

The Practice: Windshield Wipers

SUPINE CHAMPs

How to do Supine CHAMPs:

Lie flat on your back in a comfortable position.

Bend your knees to 90 degrees and place your feet flat on the floor - wider than your hips.

Move your knees slowly from side to side like a set of windshield wipers, keeping your feet on the floor.

The wider the foot stance the deeper and more active your hip stretch.

Don't do this:

Don't move through the sequence too quickly.

Don't stretch to the point of pain.

Don't forget to breathe during the movement pattern.

Do this:

Make sure your foot placement allows you to move comfortably.

Keep your hips relaxed at all times.

When you get to the sides of the "windshield wiper" try holding the stretch and relaxing the muscles.

THE BOTTOM LINE:

Keeping your hips healthy doesn't take a lot of time and energy ... but the long-lasting benefits are huge.

Mentor Memos

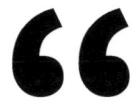

> Let yourself have some fun, challenge some rules and don't be too serious or tie yourself down before you have discovered that it's a big world out there!
>
> *Nancy Ramadan*

> Get outside, be curious, and explore.
>
> *Liz Waisberg*

> If you are lucky to have grandparents - spend time with them. Ask questions about their lives and the lessons they've learned. Once they are no longer with us, you are going to wish to have asked more and known more.
>
> *IJ Schecter*

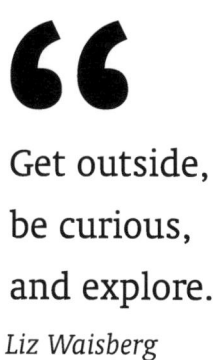

Connect The Thoughts!
Jot down notes and self-reminders here.

Mood Swinging

Own your mood and act accordingly.

Girls on periods:
I'm fine
I hate you
I love you
I want ice cream
You're cute
Screw this
Screw that

UNKNOWN

Mood Swinging

Own your mood and act accordingly.

When I was 18 I worked at my neighbourhood pharmacy in the cosmetic department. I had a knack for selling the stuff and creating beautiful displays out of gift box sets. Plus, the employee discount was a major perk.

Since the cosmetic department was female operated - hey, it was the 80's - when it came to our monthly cycle, very special attention was given.

"You 'ave your Peri-ood? - Allez chez placard!" Placard is French for the closet. This is what Francine, my French speaking supervisor used to say to me and the rest of the cosmeticians when we were menstruating.

In this closet, there were wall to wall hair colour kits that needed to be organized. Francine felt that when a woman had PMS (premenstrual syndrome), she needed to be alone.

I thought this idea was genius. Not everyone handles PMS the same, but I knew, that if I was on the sales floor, I would have literally bitten a customer's head off. I owned the mood that my period cycle brought me and I knew that my patience wouldn't be at its best. I was way better off working alone organizing hair colour kits.

Many years later, I still think about Francine and how she treated her staff. I was so lucky that I had a job and a boss that allowed me the freedom to be alone and let my emotions take over and be released, if necessary.

To this day, this is how I treat my daughter and any other female under my roof while "Aunt Flo" is visiting. Plenty of love, affection, chocolate and the licence to close your bedroom door until further notice.

Why does this happen? The hormones estrogen and progesterone go up and down throughout the menstrual cycle, which causes PMS.

Dr. Dayna Freedman MD FRCSC, Obstetrician and Gynaecologist, Fellow of the Royal College of Physicians and Surgeons of Canada has shared her thoughts on this subject.

"The hormonal changes in the menstrual cycle are marked by peaks and valleys. It is a fine balance of estrogen and progesterone. Typically, when one is rising the other is falling. At the start of the cycle it's mostly estrogen and a woman's mood tends to be good. In the second half of the cycle, progesterone is at its peak and estrogen is low. Progesterone is the hormone that drives 'moodiness'. For some people it's the 'sad' or melancholy feeling you have before your period begins. Once you get the period the estrogen begins to rise again and a 'normal' mood dominates again."

Recognize your mood and place yourself accordingly.

THE MORAL OF THE STORY:

When acknowledgment and support are given, appreciation and respect are felt which can lead to positive and rewarding returns.

Ritual: Get Your "Feel Good" Fix

Jumping rope is really good for heart health and also a great way to balance and elevate your mood.

Did you know that it's almost impossible to skip and not feel good, all at the same time?

You may think that skipping rope is something kids do at recess but there are many good reasons to understand why it offers up so many healthy and valuable benefits. Not only does it build muscle tone, coordination, balance, and cardiovascular fitness, but it can also be lots of fun and very social when you jump rope with your friends.

Skipping is also a great way to boost your mood and make you happier because it elevates your dopamine levels, which is one of the mood enhancing hormones that your body produces when you exercise. Believe it or not, it can also make you smarter (because of the way it challenges your brain), more alert, and bust fatigue!

Jumping rope can be done just about anywhere at any time. It is portable and versatile and all you need is a rope. It is a great way to burn calories, and also an excellent way to add variety to your workout routines. Both your lower and upper body are challenged to work when you jump rope and because it is a weight bearing exercise, it will help build stronger bones and muscles.

Practice: Get Your "Feel Good" Fix

SKIPPING

How to Skip:

Hold the jump rope handles in each hand and start with the rope hanging down just behind your heels.

Stand tall, feet about hip-width apart and softly engage your core.

To get the rope moving, gently rotate your arms so that the rope swings up and over your head.

As the rope makes its way down in front of you spring from your toes and jump over the rope as it moves under your feet.

Make sure you stay up on the balls of your feet.

Keep your elbows and wrists relaxed and let them move the rope.

Repeat the above steps.

Start slowly and increase your rhythm, the way you jump, and your speed when you feel comfortable.

Don't do this:

It's a lot harder than it looks so be careful not to overdo it.

Don't skip every day - give your body a chance to recuperate, take rest days.

Don't do the same thing every time you skip.

Do this:

Make sure you and your joints feel good during the workout.

Change up your workouts by hopping on both legs, one leg, alternating legs - be creative.

Change the speed of your skipping. Speed it up and slow it down.

Engage your core to protect and strengthen your hips and spine.

Jumping on a dirt surface instead of concrete will be easier on your body.

THE BOTTOM LINE:

I dare you to try and skip and not smile at the same time!

Mentor Memos

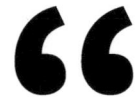

> I would give the same advice,
> my grandmother gave to me,
> "don't let other people *should* on you."
> Decide what is right in your
> own heart and do that.

Dawn Lane

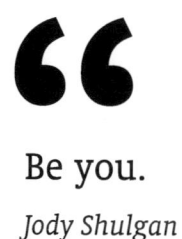

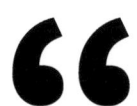

> Be you.

Jody Shulgan

> Your feelings are valid and real.
> Everyone makes mistakes,
> that's how we learn and grow.
> Listen to your heart.

Karen Gnat

Connect The Thoughts!
Jot down notes and self-reminders here.

It May Look Perfect, But It Ain't

*It looks like the
grass is greener,
but it may be fake grass
and other things, too.*

You are not defined by
an Instagram photo,
by a "like", by a comment.
That does not define you.

SELENA GOMEZ

It May Look Perfect, But It Ain't

It looks like the grass is greener, but it may be fake grass and other things, too.

Damn those posts! How did she get that angle? Why is HE at that party?

Social media is a pretty powerful platform of communication and one picture can say it all, or not. Meaning, a picture can show something "perfect" but in reality, it may be far from it.

Let's say a girl, let's call her Marcia, is sitting outside on a beautiful day, laying by a pool on a chaise lounge. Can you picture the scene? Of course you can because everyone and we mean EVERYONE has posted a picture of their legs sitting on a towel or a chair facing a body of water at some point in their lives.

You might be thinking: Why does their life look so awesome while mine sucks?

So what you see in this scene, and what you don't see could be two very different scenarios. Let me paint a picture of what you *may not* see: Marcia's parent just found out about a pile of clothes that has been sitting for weeks at the foot of her bed and the screaming match that followed was well, very loud.

A sibling just "lost" Marcia's favourite jeans that she got at a thrift store. She spent TWO WHOLE HOURS looking for this PERFECT PAIR. That one really stung, right?

Finally, Marcia's recent math test score was just posted on her school website. 47% was not the mark she intended to get. Later that day, *this is what you actually see*: Marcia lounging by her pool, looking very content.

Clearly, we don't know what is going on behind closed doors.

What *you see* looks very relaxing, decadent and perfect. But, really, YOU HAVE NO IDEA what Marcia is going through at the time of the posting. And you never will because it's none of our business.

All Marcia wants to show you is that her life is PERFECT. It's up to you if you want to believe it or not. What you see on social media may not be the truth.

THE MORAL OF THE STORY:

You will never know the whole story from an image, so to judge is not being fair. No matter what it looks like.

Ritual: The Slalom

The slalom gives you additional strength and skills because it trains your body to move sideways.

Did you know that the average person spends most of their time moving in straight lines in the forward direction?

The slalom is a very simple sideways jumping exercise that not only has a strong impact on your cardio fitness (heart and lungs), but also tones and strengthens your core, hips, and legs. It is a great way to teach the body to move and land in less familiar and different body positions. The overall effect is that walking, running, and normal day to day movements will all be much stronger and easier.

Much like skipping, side jumping also challenges your brain to think differently as it guides your body from side to side instead of the usual straight lines that you typically move in. You will be very familiar with these movements if you downhill ski, skate, dance, or do anything that involves a multi-dimensional way of moving.

Learning how to do a proper slalom jump is easy as all you need to do is move the body from side to side. It can be done just about anywhere and it needs no additional equipment or fancy set-up. You can make your workouts harder by jumping over benches that are different heights, by changing the distance of the sideways jumps, and by jumping with only one leg instead of two.

The Practice: The Slalom

THE SIDE JUMP

How to do the Side Jump:

Stand with both of your feet together on the one side of an extended line or a low bench.

Jump over the line/bench and land on both feet on the other side.

Jump back again.

Continue this side to side or zig zag movement without taking a break between jumps.

You can make the Slalom more intense by jumping on one leg instead of two.

Don't do this:

Don't make your jumps too big or wide until you feel comfortable.

Don't land your jumps heavy.

Don't do the same workout every time. Variety is key!

Do this:

Stay as light on your feet as you can.

Perform multiple jumps in rapid succession.

Vary the speed, height, and distance of your jumps as you move from side to side.

Be explosive with your jumping.

THE BOTTOM LINE:

Don't be afraid to train differently, variety is important to your overall health.

Mentor Memos

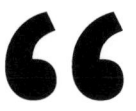

> Listen to your inner self and follow your dreams.
>
> *Lisa Kates*

> Like what YOU like, you can always unlike it. If there's a 'should' stop doing it now! Learn to hear your quiet voice.
>
> *Kev Self*

> Be brave to suck at something new.
>
> *Lisa Borden*

> Letting go of your story gives you back your power.
>
> *Andrea Scher*

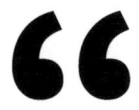

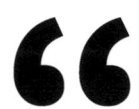

Connect The Thoughts!
Jot down notes and self-reminders here.

One Door Closes and Another Opens

When a door is locked, it may be for a reason.

**Be thankful for closed doors,
detours and roadblocks.
They protect you
from paths and places
not meant for you.**

KHLOÉ KARDASHIAN

One Door Closes and Another Opens

When a door is locked, it may be for a reason.

The time had come for my middle child to choose a high school. Since we live in a big city, we were lucky that there were 5 schools that we were interested in. Some were easier than others to get into and one, in particular, was extremely competitive to receive admittance. Of course, that was the one that my son wanted to attend.

I think it was the manicured lawns. Maybe it was the auditorium with the ginormous historical murals of notable alumni. Could it have been the perfectly orchestrated tour guides with monogrammed raincoats and umbrellas? No one really knew, except that the school was something that my son wanted to be a part of. Very badly.

An admittance test needed to be taken, so he began to study vigorously, on top of all his current subjects at school and extra curricular activities. In addition, letters of recommendation needed to be written, along with an interview.

And then there was the waiting game.

Doubting himself.

What would he do if he didn't get in?

Doubting again.

Acceptance day arrived without one for my son.

He was very sad. So sad, that he couldn't get out of bed.

"Let me just have my day of mourning." Is what he asked for. I gave it to him, along with his laptop to binge watch.

I'm all for soothing the soreness with good TV. And maybe a cookie too.

The next day, he got up from his bed and went to school. Graduated in June. In the fall, he went to the high-school that was #2 on his list. Most of his friends were attending, so that was comforting. How did he feel about it? Pretty good, but nowhere near the excitement that he would feel if he was going to THAT school.

The next four years were filled with great friends, and an enriched education to prepare him for university.

At about mid-way through his high school career, I asked him if he regretted not getting into that school. He said: "I shouldn't have gotten in - and I'm glad I didn't get in because it wasn't meant to be. I love my high school."

You would be surprised when you don't get something that you really wanted that it's actually a blessing in disguise.

THE MORAL OF THE STORY:

When you want something, you should go for it and try, regardless of whether your chances are low. If it's meant to be, it will happen. If rejection is the result - Ouch! It will sting at first. Embrace the hurt and grieve. Then move on. It may take time to realize that what you wanted wasn't meant for you. When it sinks in, you will feel the reason why you are not "there" is because you are supposed to be "here" instead.

Ritual: Standing Cat/Cow

Standing cat/cow is a gentle flow between two natural movements of your spine ... Cat (flexion) and Cow (extension).

Did you know that moving your spine daily can have a positive affect on the way you stand and carry yourself?

Your spine is the centre of your body and skeleton and it is primarily responsible for the set of your shoulders, your upright standing position, overall strength and movement, and your posture. Flexing and extending your spine can increase circulation, stimulate digestion, and generally improve how you move and feel in your body.

Standing cat/cow can be done as a part of a warm up stretch, as a way to relax your whole body, or as an exercise to manage, heal, and prevent back pain. These gentle spinal movements can also help you develop postural awareness and balance throughout your whole body.

Not only does it strengthen and stimulate your connection to your spine but also to your core muscles. It helps to open your neck, chest, shoulders, and encourages you to lengthen and deepen your inhales and exhales which can have a very positive affect on your nervous system. Standing cat/cow can help you to release stress, and calm and centre your thoughts when you're dealing with life's everyday ups and downs.

Practice: Standing Cat/Cow

SPINAL MOBILITY

How to do Standing Cat/Cow:

Stand in a comfortable upright position with your feet about hip width apart.

Place your head in a neutral position and keep your neck relaxed.

Gently move into standing Cat Pose: Exhale as you drop your chin down toward your chest.

Allow your shoulders to round forward.

Slowly tuck your tailbone between your legs and round your middle spine.

As you exhale move into Cow Pose: Draw your arms and shoulders back and move your chest forward and into an open heart position.

Tilt your head and look upward.

Tilt your tailbone out and behind you.

Gently and slowly repeat the movement from Cat to Cow and back again.

Don't do this:

Don't move too quickly between cat and cow.

Don't raise your head too high and strain your neck.

Don't drop down into your shoulders.

Do this:

Stay connected to your breathing from one posture to the other.

Make sure you inhale as you move into Cow.

Make sure you exhale as you move into Cat.

Keep your movement comfortable and in your spine.

Connect yourself to your core.

THE BOTTOM LINE:

Proud confident posture is a product of a healthy and flexible spine.

Mentor Memos

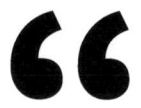

> Stop spending
> so much time worrying
> about the future
> and enjoy the moment.

Kathleen Sommerville

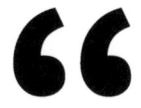

> In life, it will be YOUR fear that stops you,
> when you could have done it.
> Fear looks like:
> "that's too hard",
> "I'm not good enough".
> The opposite of fear, is LOVE.
> Love looks like:
> "it's hard, but I'll get it".
> "I'm not good enough now,
> but I'll get better".
> Love always wins.
> Choose love, and you'll always win.

Rich Knox

Connect The Thoughts!
Jot down notes and self-reminders here.

14

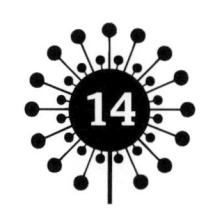

Great-FULL

*Gratitude practice,
a healthy habit
that we all need to do.
Especially now.*

I don't have to have
extraordinary moments
to find happiness -
it's right there in front of me
if I'm paying attention and
practicing gratitude.

BRENÉ BROWN

Great-FULL

Gratitude practice, a healthy habit that we all need to do. Especially now.

No, it's not a typo. It should be written this way: grateful. When I take a moment to push away all distractions, and really focus on what is in front of me, I find myself appreciating the littlest things that bring me pure joy.

It's gratitude that is taken to a whole new level and I'm calling it "Great-FULL". For instance, I am feeling great-FULL for a pair of socks.

I recently bought a pair of cotton socks from Soulmate Socks - you know the ones that are super soft, with funky fabulous patterns? Anyway, they are the most comfy, beautiful and fun socks that I own and I reserve them for Sundays.

Sunday is my work and prep day for the week. Not the most exciting glamorous day, that's for sure. More like a "chore-day". Laundry. A food shop. Prepping meals.

I'm all about making my environment a little more special and decadent when I have things I gotta get done. Even when I don't want to do them.

It makes the process way more bearable and most importantly, enjoyable.

As I get dressed for the day and open my sock drawer, a rush of glee fills my soul as my eyes dash directly to the super cool and cozy Soulmate Socks. I love how they stand out in my sea of mundane regular socks that I wear during the week.

As I slip them on, I let my toes wiggle around to feel the soft cotton. My feet feel as "snug as a bug" in them. After getting dressed, I look at myself in the mirror and smile. My feet look so cute! I think to myself as I turn on my heel and begin to putter around the house.

My gratitude cup runneth over a pair of socks.

Imagine that.

And then there's that little screen that I am guilty for carrying around in my hand. I can't imagine being interrupted by my smartphone while putting on my socks as it would totally rob every moment of my gratitude.

And that's what makes the practice of being great-FULL challenging.

In order to feel great-FULL, you need to have no distractions and be present. To appreciate the moment that something amazing is happening.

Whether it's putting on a pair of socks, taking that first sip of coffee or, my favourite one: holding someone's hand. Someone that's special to you.

Nothing beats that one.

THE MORAL OF THE STORY:

Appreciating and being great-FULL of the little things in life is so much more appreciated without any distractions.

The more you are great-FULL for, the more happiness you will have in your life.

Ritual: Feeling Good About Me

Self-gazing is a beautiful and enriching way to deeply connect to your inner self.

Did you know that there is way more to you than just the way you look?

There are studies that show that self-gazing daily can greatly reduce stress, and at the same time increase your gratitude and self-compassion. Remember, gratitude and appreciation build self-confidence and self-confidence leads to self-kindness, so don't be afraid to gaze deeply into your own eyes.

Gazing into a mirror gives you the opportunity to look beyond your appearance and physical traits and it encourages you to face your inner emotions and any unrest you might be dealing with. It will also help you identify and understand your self-judgment and counter these feelings with self-compassion and love.

When you begin the process of self-gazing it can make you feel uncomfortable, especially if you're not used to spending time standing in front of a mirror, looking into your own eyes. It is important to realize that this process can hold the key to you understanding and appreciating the depths of your true self. Regardless of the awkward feelings you might have when you first start doing this. Give it a try for a week and you will see that eventually it gets easier and way more comfortable.

Practice: Feeling Good About Me

SELF-GAZING

How To Self-Gaze:

Set up a mirror in a quiet place that is free of distractions.

Angle the mirror so that you can comfortably gaze directly into your own eyes.

Close your eyes and slowly bring yourself into the moment by connecting to your breathing.

Allow your whole body to relax.

When you feel relaxed open your eyes and look at yourself in the mirror.

Continue to pay attention to your breathing as it will help you stay centred.

Pay attention to the thoughts that come into your mind.

Let your thoughts go to wherever they might, but continue to gaze into your eyes from a place of love and kindness.

Don't do this:

Don't focus on things that you dislike about yourself.

Don't focus on your flaws.

Don't be critical or judgmental.

Do this:

Visualize your breath releasing your dislikes.

Observe whatever negative feelings come up and then let them go.

Pay attention to the emotions in your eyes and on your face.

Gaze at yourself with kindness and reflection.

THE BOTTOM LINE:
Gazing into your own eyes daily fosters self-appreciation, GRATITUDE, compassion, and self-love.

Mentor Memos

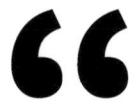

"

Having balance in life
is a key to happiness and joy.
Make sure to make time
for family, friendships,
extra-curricular activities,
hobbies along with school work.
Continuously explore new hobbies,
courses, activities and see
what brings you joy in life.

Govind Kilambi

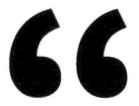

"

Don't be so worried
about making mistakes.
Everyone is too concerned
about their own
to worry about yours.

Shannon Coleclough

Connect The Thoughts!
Jot down notes and self-reminders here.

Salad Master

*There is more than
one way to
eat your greens!*

For the first time since 2007, the FDA has approved a new device to treat obesity. The amazing breakthrough is called a vegetable.

CONAN O'BRIEN

Salad Master

There is more than one way to eat your greens!

If you're one of those people who eat vegetables all the time - great! Good for you. You can stop reading now and go make yourself a salad.

Then there's the rest of us!

We can only imagine your frustration with the continuous banter of people telling you to EAT YOUR VEGGIES.

And this book is all about taking care of your body, mind, and soul. How could we not include a favourite recipe, that is not only healthy but yummy? This recipe is especially for those of you who:

*Gag at the sight of anything green.

*Love chocolate

*Are open to trying anything once (oh, come on! It will be fun!)

Before we post the sneakiest, tastiest recipe right here on this page, we first have to tell you WHY you need to eat your greens.

*Protects your body from disease (really - go Google it)

*Helps you poop (we can witness this is true)

*Gives you energy (who's up for a game of basketball?)

Good enough reasons, right?

Now onto the recipe.

Chocolate Sneaky Spinach Smoothie

1 cup of milk (almond, cow's milk, or oat milk)

1/2 cup of frozen spinach
(kale also works and NO, you won't taste it - trust us!)

1/2 banana

1 tbsp nut butter of choice (seed butter works well too)

1 tbsp chocolate protein powder or cacao powder

A handful of ice

One dash or two of cinnamon

Blend, baby, blend!

Taste it. Does it need a little more of this? Or that? Go ahead and add it in - this recipe is not set in stone; you make the rules because you are the chef - and the one drinking it!

THE MORAL OF THE STORY:

Your daily dose of greens keeps your body running smoothly, with an added dose of energy! The magic nutrients in greens protect your body from disease.

Ritual: The Lunge Matrix

There is more than one "best and healthy" way to move your body!

Did you know that your body is a multi-dimensional moving machine?

You typically move your body in straights lines, the sidewalks and roads have taught you to do this. The equipment in gyms, treadmills, stair climbers, and stationary bikes, teach you to move in straight lines as well. When you go for a run outdoors it's more straight lines ... It's the quickest, healthiest, and most efficient way for you to move your body, right?

Actually NO! Humans ... and that includes you, are notorious for finding the easiest way to get things done. It's our default setting even though it's not always the healthiest way to do things in the long term. Healthy full-body movement is way more than moving in straight lines.

So what is the healthiest way to move anyway?

Forward, backward, from side-to-side, up, down, on a 45 degree angle, rotationally, and here's the clincher, in "combinations" of all of the above! If this is confusing to you, watch a young child move, they're up and over and twisting and turning, and on the floor, and rolling around ... you get the picture? Ideally, we don't want to lose that sense of childlike play when we are moving our bodies.

The lunge matrix is a series of lunges and squats that move you in all directions. This sequence strengthens the way you are designed to move naturally. Not only does it offer you greater spatial awareness and movement freedom, but also strength, balance, versatility and resilience.

Practice: The Lunge Matrix

LUNGE SQUAT SEQUENCE

How to do the Lunge Squat Sequence:

Start in an upright standing position.

After each of the following moves, return to centre.

Step your right foot forward (lunge) bending both knees to about 90 degrees.

Step your right foot forward at a 45-degree angle to the right (lunge).

Step your right foot to the right side (squat) bending both knees to about 90 degrees.

Step your right foot back at a 45-degree angle to the right (squat).

Step your right foot backward (lunge) bending both knees to about 90 degrees.

Repeat this same sequence using your left foot.

One complete Lunge Matrix is all moves on both sides.

Don't do this:

Don't make your steps too big or you will be uncomfortable.

Don't create knee pain during the movements.

Don't forget to breathe.

Do this:

Try doing this on the grass for less stability.

Use your arms to help with balance.

Keep your head up and your shoulders proud.

THE BOTTOM LINE:

Multidimensional movement teaches us to be capable, confident, and free in our bodies.

Mentor Memos

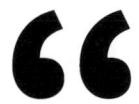

"

Seek out ways you can add
your greatest value and
be your best self.
Always.
Because that is what
the world needs from you.
Nothing good ever comes from looking
for the easiest way through.
Take the stairs.

Richard Carmichael

"

Be kind and
go vegan!
It's the best choice
for animals, the planet
and yourself!

Oren Epstein

Connect The Thoughts!
Jot down notes and self-reminders here.

It's All Perspective

Change your way of thinking, which will in turn change your view.

**It's not what you look at
that matters,
it's what you see.**

HENRY DAVID THOREAU

It's All Perspective

Change your way of thinking, which will in turn change your view.

Back in 1999, when I gave birth to my eldest son Josh, I looked up at the nurse and asked "Now what?"

Needless to say, I figured it out. Today, Josh is a 21-year-old university student and is soaring physically and emotionally. Heck, my husband and I even like him, too.

As I write this, it is March 19th, 2020 and like the rest of the world, we have to follow a long list of strict COVID-19 rules. Josh said to me this morning. "How long will this last?" My mind went directly to the time when I gave birth to him.

When Josh was first born, I didn't sleep for four straight months.

When I say I didn't sleep, it means that I didn't sleep well. I was woken up at least three times during the night to feed him which took about one to two hours each time. Every baby is different and I happened to fall into a routine that involved feeding, burping, maybe changing a diaper and rocking him back to sleep. Each day when I would see the sunrise, I would say to myself, "How long is this going to last?"

Let's take a look at the word *this*.

Replace it with the situation "du jour" in this case, it's COVID-19.

I look back on that time with honour. I look at Josh and I am amazed at what I helped grow.

While I was going through it, it was hard. It wasn't fun and I needed it to stop.

But would I do it again?

In a heartbeat. I needed to do my job as a mother - as best as I knew how.

And now I'm doing the best that I can for my family and I during this pandemic. Even though it's hard. I am missing a lot.

At the time of publication, this pandemic has surpassed my four-month comparison to my newborn's sleepless nights. I still have a long list of things that I miss. I'm sure you can list a few, or 36.

Back then, I decided that I wasn't going to look at how long this would last. I was going to take one day at a time and be the best mother I could be. There were things that I could control, (the food I ate, the people I surrounded myself with) and things that I couldn't control (sleep, sleep and more sleep).

And now, 21 years later, even though the situation is different, I am going to take my own advice, once again and change my perspective so I can get through these extraordinary times.

THE MORAL OF THE STORY:

Challenging times are challenging for a reason. It's all about the approach and attitude. Focus on what you can do to get through these challenging days, which only brings you resilience and wisdom.

Ritual: Gaze Shifting

There are four stages of growth when we are exposed to something new in our lives. Confusion ... Discomfort ... Adaptation ... Improvement.

Did you know that asking a simple question or being inquisitive is the first stage of the process of understanding something new?

Our lives are full of new situations! They crop up every single day and the process of learning and growing are the basis for our ever expanding intelligence and wisdom. Simple situations usually involve a very fast and easy learning process and more complex situations might take much more time and energy.

For example, think about the simple act of rotating your neck and moving your head from side to side. Something that we've done daily since we were born. Now think about that complicated math problem that you had to sit and stew on, the one that caused you to throw your hands up in the air and get really dramatic about.

This process of moving from "not knowing" to "knowing", whether it be physical or mental is the basis for our very existence, our survival, and growth. Imagine where Josh would be today if his mother threw up her hands and said, "You know what? It's too hard. I can't do it!" His outcome would be very, very different.

There are four basic stages of learning and growing when we are exposed to something new. The first stage is confusion ... simply because it is new and we have no prior knowledge of the situation. The second stage is that it usually makes us feel uncomfortable. The third stage is our natural tendency to adapt to this new situation so that we can evolve, grow, thrive, and survive. And finally, the fourth stage is when we notice our improvement!

Gaze shifting is a natural and healthy movement pattern that is designed to improve the way your neck moves. Rotating your neck daily promotes blood flow, lubricates your joints, and challenges your brain!

Practice: Gaze Shifting

NECK ROTATIONS

How to rotate your neck:

Turn your head and look over your left shoulder.

Turn your head back to the front.

Turn your head and look over your right shoulder.

Return to the front and repeat.

Don't do this:

Don't make your movements so big that they cause pain.

Don't move too quickly.

Don't tense up your shoulders.

Do this:

Move slowly and mindfully.

Close your eyes so that you're not distracted.

Keep your breathing very relaxed.

THE BOTTOM LINE:

If you use it ... you won't lose it!

Mentor Memos

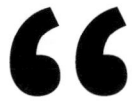

> "You might not know it now, but hygiene is a huge indicator of how you present yourself. It is something that you alone have control over. Being aware of the products you use and how they affect your body and health will, in turn, have a direct impact on our planet. Choose your products wisely."
>
> Brian Phillips

> If adversity and mental health challenges come knocking on your door, know that your relationship to these challenges will matter a lot more than the challenges themselves. Perspective is everything.
>
> Ryan Golt

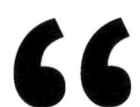

Connect The Thoughts!
Jot down notes and self-reminders here.

Just Keep Cleaning ...
Just Keep Cleaning

Housekeeping for your soul.

**If you avoid conflict
to keep the peace,
you start a war
within yourself.**

UNKNOWN

Just Keep Cleaning... Just Keep Cleaning

Housekeeping for your soul.

We're not talking brooms, buckets and bleach here.

Your life is filled with people, projects, jobs, and expectations.

Along for the ride there will be uncomfortable confrontations.

100% guaranteed.

Most people are on "auto pilot" and go through their days avoiding facing things that get in their way. This unfortunately can build up tension between people, kind of like dust on a shelf.

Before long, the dust may get too thick, and then you need the help of a heavy duty cleaner, along with someone to handle the machinery to chisel away at the many layers of "dirt".

"I hate it when you leave your wet towel on the floor. Pick. It. Up."

"_____" (No response, but it was heard!)

It seems as if this problem has been going on for a while. Watch how it explodes.

"We share a bathroom! Pick it up! Mooooommmmm!"

"_____" Mom's reaction. She doesn't want to get involved.

While your family members can be a great support system, they can also really grind your gears. If a sibling, or anyone in your life repeatedly does something that bugs you, and you don't say anything, your anger will just get increasingly worse, day after day, week after week and then the inevitable will happen. You will yell.

Yelling is a great tension release and it's a completely normal reaction when you're totally peeved. However, it is incredibly unproductive. When you yell at someone, all that is heard is noise.

The next time you get upset, walk away. Relieve your tension by going for a walk and do the exercise on the next page. You will then be able to gather your thoughts and be able to express them in a clear and calm manner.

Like this: "When you leave your towel on the floor, it really bothers me. It's also my bathroom, too. We all have to do our part in keeping the bathroom clean. Put your used towel on the hook. Plus, by not leaving it on the floor, you are keeping the towel clean, which saves us water. So you are not only helping to keep the bathroom clean, you are helping the planet."

Offering a quick solution, with added benefits, without yelling, will help release the frustrated feelings. Even if no positive results occur, the fact that the complainer did the very best to deal with the problem, will have a positive effect for the level of frustration.

THE MORAL OF THE STORY:

Deal with problems as best as you can. Even if your desired results don't follow, something else may. By sharing what is bothering you, it prevents build up which can tamper with the current relationship, going forward. Continuously expressing your feelings helps create a stronger and productive relationship that needs less "fixing".

Ritual: The Helicopter

Uncomfortable problems most often get worse when you avoid them.

Did you know that you are naturally hardwired to avoid confrontation even if you know that it will cause you future problems?

When you are bothered by a situation like someone leaving a towel on the bathroom floor, you have options. Do you live with it? Do you express your frustration? Is there an easy solution? How do you address the problem and speak your peace? Do you just let it go because it's easier than expressing yourself?

Your physical body is designed the same way. You naturally find the easiest way to move your body even if it is bad for you in the long-term. It's an energy conservation thing and you are built to use energy only when you need it. Take for example, exercising or going for a run. You have to push yourself because it's not something you want to do naturally. If you think about it, running was something that ancient man did to either escape danger or hunt animals for food, he did not run for fun.

The problem associated with this is that when you stop using your joints and muscles they weaken and become unstable and less capable of doing what they were designed to do. This is especially evident in the aging population. Everyone has witnessed someone struggle with basic movement like sitting or standing, going up or down a flight of stairs, putting their socks on.

So in order to age well you need to partake in multi-dimensional full body movements on a daily basis. You need to keep your body strong and your joints happy and healthy so that you have them for the rest of your life. You need to show up for yourself everyday.

Rotating your spine daily promotes blood flow, joint lubrication, and challenges your brain to remember how to do it well. Much like Gaze-Shifting, The Helicopter is an easy and healthy movement pattern that is designed to improve the way your middle spine, shoulders, and hips move.

Practice: The Helicopter

MID SPINE ROTATIONS

How to do Mid Spine Rotations:

Stand in a comfortable position with your feet a little wider than your hips.

Extend your arms out and down to the sides of your body.

Start twisting your head, shoulders, and mid body to the left letting your arms swing out and away from your body.

Twist your head, shoulders, and mid body to the right and let your arms move the same way.

Your arms should move like a helicopter or a tether ball.

Repeat the movement fluidly back and forth.

Don't do this:

Don't over rotate your spine.

Don't hunch your spine.

Don't forget to breathe.

Do this:

Keep your breathing relaxed during the rotations.

Let your arms swing in a relaxed manner.

Let your hands gently slap your body at the end of the rotation.

THE BOTTOM LINE:

Your health tomorrow depends on your care today.

Mentor Memos

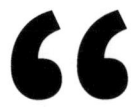

> Make your default setting to help -
> be willing to help anyone at any time -
> especially before you are asked.

Rob Storm

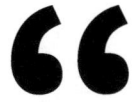

> No matter what time of life,
> find a way to do the healthy
> activities you love in groups.
> You'll find your friends
> are already there.

Colleen Kavanagh

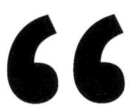

> You are
> beautiful baby,
> know your worth.

Lisa Binns

Connect The Thoughts!
Jot down notes and self-reminders here.

Letting Go

*As you make a change,
you never know
what you will reinvent.*

**We need to keep moving forward,
opening new doors,
and doing new things, because
we're curious and curiosity keeps
leading us down new paths.**

WALT DISNEY

Letting Go

As you make a change, you never know what you will reinvent.

March 16th, 2020. The COVID-19 Lockdown was in full force. Schools, restaurants and gyms closed their doors. Social gatherings, including national sport games, were cancelled. Big chain grocery stores had lineups as far as the eye can see and people were afraid to run out of toilet paper.

Before the pandemic, no matter how chaotic life got, I always counted on going to my gym where I enjoyed the sport of weight lifting. I suddenly could no longer go there anymore because a gym became a place where the virus could spread.

I had to let go of my regular routine and begin something different.

Making that lifestyle change was not easy. I had specific exercises with certain machines that I couldn't do at home. Concerns began to flood my mind. Would my home workouts be challenging enough? Could I be self-motivated without being at my gym?

I had no idea, but I had to begin to find out.

On that first day of my new routine, I opened my front door and breathed in the fresh air. I felt the warm sunshine on my face and admired the beautiful shade of blue the sky was showing off that day.

I clicked on the songs from my playlist that motivated me and I began to run.

When I returned home, my head sunk down and I quickly realized that there were no barbells waiting for me, nor any of my friends at the gym to share what rep I was on.

Out of the corner of my eye I saw a huge brick that acted as a weight to keep my yard door open.

I lifted it up and it felt as heavy as the weight I typically used at the gym and I began to utilize it for a series of exercises. Was I able to completely replicate my gym routine with this brick? Not really. But it became a close second, which was good enough for me.

Since that day in March, my home workout routine has expanded way beyond that large brick. It wasn't easy to change my habit, but I let it go and created something new, which I think is pretty powerful.

THE MORAL OF THE STORY:

Letting go of something allows you to let in something else. With a little imagination, you can let go of what you're used to and create something totally new and exciting.

Letting go enables you to become adaptable to change, which is inevitable.

Ritual: Off-Road-Speed-Play

When we change we grow.

Did you know that you are not supposed to be a creature of habit?

Your body thrives on change. Your health and longevity depend on it. But at the same time you think you thrive on routine. Routines are easy, they are predictable and don't really challenge us either physically or mentally. They allow us to be lazy, and boy do we like lazy. An important thing to remember is that when you repeat the same thing over and over you will most likely achieve the same results over and over.

Being forced to change and give up something that you enjoy is not the end of the world. In fact when you interrupt habits and force yourself to do something new and different you are challenging yourself to be adaptable. This adaptability is the key to growth not only in your body but also for your mind! Changing your gym routine requires effort and these efforts will most certainly decrease boredom, boost your mood, and support your mental health.

Off-Road-Speed-Play is the perfect way to build change and adaptability into your workouts. No two runs will ever be the same so you can be sure that you will be in a constant state of learning and adapting. Trail running is much more fun than running on the road, and at the same time puts less stress on your body but will challenge your brain to wake up and learn new and exciting ways to move.

Also, getting out of the gym and working out in nature has so many benefits! It will boost your immune system, you will get a big dose of vitamin D, burn more calories, and release more "feel good" hormones. As a result, you will probably work out longer and harder. So get outside! Explore, play, and enjoy the vastness and challenges of the outdoor gym.

Practice: Off-Road-Speed-Play

TRAIL RUNNING

How to Trail Run:

You don't need specific equipment to trail run.

Pick a relatively flat and easy trail if you are a beginner.

Make sure the trail is either an out-and-back or is a loop and has you starting and finishing at the same spot.

You can choose more challenging terrain as you become stronger and more familiar with the trails.

Don't do this:

Don't make it about speed, pace yourself.

Don't be afraid to break into a walk if you need some recovery time.

Don't overtrain, build up your workouts over time.

Do this:

Make sure you stay connected to your body and the terrain.

Do a warm-up walk before you start to run.

Enjoy the beautiful offerings of Mother Nature!

THE BOTTOM LINE:

Being adaptable will lead you to your greatest successes!

Mentor Memos

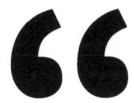

❝

Enjoy life and don't worry so much.
99 percent of what we worry about
never happens. So try to live in
the present moment as much as possible,
not worrying about what has just happened,
or what's about to happen.
Everything has a way of falling into place,
especially when you replace worry
with feelings of calm and trust,
and know that where you are right now,
is exactly where you need to be.

Judy Librach

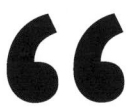

❝

Believe in yourself,
you are important,
and never give up
on your dreams.

Maria Biber

Connect The Thoughts!
Jot down notes and self-reminders here.

Whoa!

Stop that galloping horse.
Stop for just a moment.
And think.

Sometimes it's the journey that teaches you a lot about your destination.

DRAKE

Whoa

Stop that galloping horse. Stop for just a moment. And think.

Got a topic you want information on? You know you can get your answers as fast as you can type. Research project on Winston Churchill? Check. Nothing on TV? That's so 2010. Watch how a person can eat 10,000 calories in a day. Not only fascinating, but fast.

This is all wonderful and easy and it seems to be working really well for everyone. Nothing like being on the receiving end of the internet.

I can see your eyes roll. The idea of waiting for something can be viewed as so boring. I mean, what's there to do? Sit. And. Wait.

And?

Wait for it.

Whoa. Meaning, STOP, for just a moment. And think.

Think about what happened yesterday. What you said to so and so. How did it make you feel. Think about HOW you want your history paper to look like before you google Churchill. You need to WAIT and say WHOA before making any major decisions. As you would make your coffee or tea, you need to take the time to brew your ideas.

It's all about taking the time to process the situation before you arrive at your final destination.

Let's try this fun exercise: During the colder months, when you come home from being outside and your lips are the same colour as a blueberry, take some time out to enjoy a cup of hot chocolate.

Put your electronic device aside.

Choose a quiet place in your home for just you. Hold the cup with two hands and feel the warmth radiate through the palms of your hands. Inhale the aroma of the chocolate and then exhale. Take that first sip and savour the cocoa flavour.

The beauty of this exercise, is that it can be done with just about anything. Choose your poison! Tea, water or the scent of a candle. But don't drink the candle wax! ;)

By taking the time to say whoa. To stop and think, gives your body a chance to reduce stress and clear your mind. When you are in this state, the possibilities of where you can go have no limits.

THE MORAL OF THE STORY:

It may seem counterintuitive, but by saying "whoa" and stopping all of the whirlwind to-do lists and things that are racing around in your head will allow you to be more productive. You will get a chance to gather your thoughts and think about priorities. You will have the ability to reduce anxiety and stress, improve learning, and improve sleep. Skills that are so needed for you to live your best life.

Ritual: Start by Stopping

Start by Stopping is the simple act of bringing yourself to a place of complete stillness, for just a moment, by concentrating on your inhales and exhales.

Did you know that starting a task with a moment of complete stillness gives you a chance to clear away all of the muddle in your head?

Start by Stopping gives you the chance to bring yourself into the moment. It encourages you to root yourself in breath and to overview your current state of being. It builds sharper concentration, enhances memory, and releases stress. All of these things are known to improve your mental health.

The next time you are preparing to study for a test and experience "exam jitters", pause for a couple of seconds and consider what you are about to do and its significance in the greater picture of your everyday life. The simple act of studying builds "mental muscle" and "resilience". It also builds confidence, self-esteem, and strengthens your ability to remember things.

Even the most mundane tasks, like walking up or down a flight of stairs, or brushing your teeth, have great impact when you stop and truly think about what you are doing. When you take the time to "Start by Stopping" as you make your way through your day and life, from your morning habits to your school work, to sharing a meal with your family and friends, you are stopping to experience a richer more mindful connection and experience to your own actions.

Practice: Start by Stopping

MINDFUL CONNECTION

How to practice Mindful Connection:

Find a comfortable seated or standing position.

Close or lower your eyes.

Notice the natural and gentle rhythm of your breath and deepen your connection to it.

Bring your body and mind to a place of complete stillness.

If your thoughts start to wander, gently bring yourself back to breath.

Don't do this:

Don't connect or create distraction with music and podcasts.

Don't be judgmental if you struggle to quiet the mind.

Don't be impatient with the process of stillness.

Do this:

Pay close attention to the sensations that arise in your body like your heartbeat and breath.

Take in your environment through all of your senses.

Use your breathing as your primary way to connect to the self.

THE BOTTOM LINE:

Starting tasks with moments of stillness will bring greater connection and value to your day to day life.

Mentor Memos

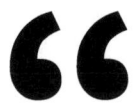

> Ask more questions. Seek help from experts, not just your teachers but people who have gone before you in all walks of life. Then work through the offerings, answers and advice with your peers to fully understand it (what does it all mean?) then improve it - if you can.

John Mason

> Music is
> a way in and
> a way out.

Noa Daniel

> Time is not a renewable resource so use it well.

Dayna Freedman

Connect The Thoughts!
Jot down notes and self-reminders here.

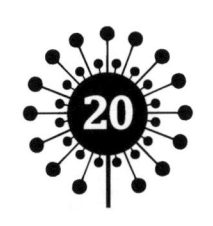

The Magic of Failure

It's humiliating and painful, but you need it in your life.

**Failure is success
in progress.**

ALBERT EINSTEIN

The Magic of Failure

It's humiliating and painful, but you need it in your life.

I love to keep all things organized! Knowing where everything is and where everyone goes makes my heart sing. Especially when it's all written down somewhere, like on a calendar.

I had a generic family wall calendar that I used religiously, but I felt frustrated having to rewrite recurring activities over and over again. Swimming on Mondays, flag football on Wednesdays. I was missing an easy, fast and smart solution to family organization.

Necessity is the mother of invention, so, I invented a wall calendar that was unique, simple and clear. It carried a unique design that enabled the user to write down a school year of activities in a flash.

I've always been one to take the leap. To go for it. Being brave is one of my strengths and so I moved forward, without hesitation.

Even though the rising popularity of digital calendars and smart phones were beginning to take the stage at that time, wall calendars still existed, and I was determined to create the best one in the world.

I did not have a proper business plan, nor did I research the calendar market properly. Help from different people was thrown at me from various resources. Some were very helpful and generous. Some were not.

Despite the challenges, the calendar was loved by many, won a few awards and was featured on television, too.

Some barked that I was living in the dark ages as they waved their smartphone in my face. To this day, I feel that both have their own merit, and there's something to be said for writing things down.

I continued to persevere for several more years until I decided to throw in the towel and stop production. My soul couldn't take the chase anymore and I was mentally exhausted.

The term I use for this calendar project is FAIL. This stands for First Attempt In Learning. There is a laundry list of things I learned that I take with me everywhere.

Although it was a painful and costly process, I wouldn't trade the experience I went through for anything. Because of what it taught me.

THE MORAL OF THE STORY:

Trying something out of the ordinary that stretches your bravery and perseverance is something to be proud of. Even if you FAIL, you still tried and you will take the lessons with you forever.

Ritual: I Can't Do This!

The definition of failure is being unsuccessful or not achieving a desired action. However ...

Did you know that success is built on failure?

You will never meet a successful person who can honestly admit that they haven't failed ... and probably multiple times! Failure happens, and you need to embrace that it will, and that you will have your fair share of it. Another thing that you need to understand is that from each failure, you learn two very important lessons. One, that there was at least one reason you failed; and two, that you can always learn and recover from your failures.

You can only understand failure by having experienced what success feels like and, the only way you can understand success is by knowing what it feels like to fail. Take a moment to chew on that. It's like "hot" has no meaning without knowing what "cold" feels like, and cold is nothing without hot. So failure is a very natural and normal part of your everyday life as are your successes.

We also know that failure is often the byproduct of a lack of persistence, tenacity, preparation, and practice. All of which are valuable life skills that we develop and learn. Another challenging thing you need to do is to hold onto and remember your past failures for they will most definitely be one of your biggest learnings that you carry forward.

The One Hundreds is an exercise that not only builds tenacity and strength, but also gives you a greater sense of grounding, stability, and foundation ... all of which your future successes will be built upon. This is the perfect sequence because the first time you do it, and possibly the second and third, you will most certainly fail. Perhaps you will get to 30 or if you're lucky 40. Eventually 40 will feel easier and you'll fail at 60. Practising 60 will take you to 80 and before you know it you will realize the success of 100 deep squats. Your success will be the byproduct of patience, persistence, and focus, and of course your ability to embrace and use failure to motivate you toward your ultimate goal of being successful.

Good luck and enjoy your success but don't forget to embrace your struggles!

Practice: I Can't Do This!

THE ONE HUNDREDS

How to do The One Hundreds:

Start in an upright standing position with your feet a little wider than your hips.

Raise your arms to shoulder height straight out in front of you (for balance).

Slowly sit down as though you are sitting into a chair.

Stop when your hips are slightly higher than your knees.

With control move up about six inches and return to the lower position.

Do this 100 times!

Don't do this:

Don't squat too deeply until you're ready.

Don't forget to breathe.

Don't give in until you feel failure.

Do this:

Make sure you keep your movements to about six inches up and down.

Stay in a deep squat for as long as you can.

Use your core to protect your back and to keep shoulders strong and stable.

THE BOTTOM LINE:

Struggle leads to great growth.

Mentor Memos

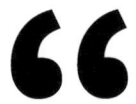

> Travel and experience the world
> outside of what you know.
> The school of life is a great way to learn.
>
> Always have a curious mind,
> especially when you are met
> by what may seem like a road block.
> It will most likely only be an obstacle to
> creatively find a way around,
> or to even change your mind about.
> You will always learn
> something in the process.
>
> Lead with a compassionate heart.
> Leaning in and helping others is
> always more gratifying than not.
> You will get the same in return
> when you are in need.

Marla Gold

Connect The Thoughts!
Jot down notes and self-reminders here.

21

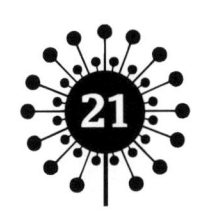

Find Your People.
Know Your People.

Choose your friends wisely.

**Be who you are
and say how you feel,
because those who mind
don't matter,
and those who matter
don't mind.**

DR. SEUSS

Find Your People. Know Your People.

Choose your friends wisely.

I pass by them. I watch from afar. It's so appealing that it makes me question my world. Am I meant to be here? Am I meant to be there?

I eavesdrop on what they are doing and it sounds so enticing. I wonder what it would be like to be with them.

He asks me after English class.

"I know we are friends with different people, but I still want to go to prom with you."

Here's my chance and I accept. Even though I will be away from my people, for a short while, I still want to go there.

I also want to be with him too, because he's my friend. Besides, I don't want a group of people to get in the way of who I was going to prom with.

Prom day arrives.

Dress is good. My hair is the way I envisioned it. I'm ready. I'm so curious to experience being with these people.

We go to the "Pre."

My eyes dart around. They look me up and down with fierce and strong stares. My date puts his arm around my waist, which I like. It makes me feel safe. Although I still feel uncomfortable, I don't want to leave.

I stand around and listen. I say a few words. Laugh.

Was I supposed to laugh?

"How did you get here?" I am bluntly asked.

"She's with me." My date defends. I smile. My heart pounds.

We stay for a little while longer and I find myself looking out the window, thinking of whom I left behind.

We push through the large doors to the hall and I see them, standing in a huddle. They see me and a rush of comfort fills my soul. This is where I belong.

Even though it looked like fun, that world is not meant for me.

THE MORAL OF THE STORY:

Before you join a different friend group, accept that you may not be happy with them. Find friends that make you feel complete and supported. Having friends that you love and accept you as you are will help you get through life's obstacles.

Ritual: The Big Squeeze

We offer hugs to others as a source of comfort when they are sad and in pain. We look for hugs from others for the same reasons ... they are as good to give as they are to receive!

Did you know that hugs have been proven to make us feel better in good times and bad?

A hug can send the "I care about you, you matter, and you are not alone" message. In fact, the warmth of your embrace is more nourishing to your soul than food.

Have you ever experienced a time in your life when you've been angry or upset and someone offered you a big hug and the way you felt quickly disappeared? Can you also feel someone's angst disappear when you offer your embrace? Most everybody understands the immediate, long lasting, and comforting effects of a hug.

The science of hugging goes way beyond the warm feelings that you get when you hold someone in your arms. A hug offers you a sense of belonging and support, helps you deal with pain and unpleasant circumstances, and raises oxytocin levels which makes you feel happier and less stressed. Giving someone a hug can not only reduce their stress but can also reduce your stress as well, a beautiful two way flow of energy.

A couple of other things to consider when you are hugging someone else - the timing and the contact. You need to be intuitive as to what the other person needs so that you don't end the hug too early or hold on too long or too tight. To avoid an awkward situation let the person you are hugging indicate what they want by how hard they squeeze you and for how long they feel comfortable, if their hug is soft then hug them back softly. One important consideration is to not impose a hug on someone if they don't look like they are prepared to hug you back. In situations like these it is probably best to back off.

The Big Squeeze is a beautiful exercise that can show intimacy, vulnerability, and display great affection and care.

Practice: The Big Squeeze

THE HUG CHALLENGE

How to do the Hug Challenge:

Approach the person you are going to hug with kind feelings.

Lean forward and put your two arms around the person.

Be genuine and positive with your energy.

Press your body gently into theirs.

Smile at them when you let go.

Don't do this:

Don't hug someone if they don't want to be hugged.

Don't embrace the person too tightly.

Don't hug the person too long.

Do this:

Tell the person that you care about them.

Let the person know that everything is going to be okay.

If appropriate, add a gentle comforting caress on the shoulder.

THE BOTTOM LINE:

You need four daily hugs to survive, and 12 to thrive ...
so give and get as many hugs as possible.

Mentor Memos

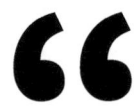

"

The point of this time in your life is not to
have everything figured out or to try to do so.
The focus needs to be on exploring who
you truly are (self-development),
what this world has to offer
(opening your perspective),
understanding your unique gifts, talents, and
natural tendencies because these are often
the guide to what inspires you to live
meaningfully. Surround yourself with things,
and people that inspire or motivate you
to express yourself as you are and,
most importantly, keep in mind that all heroes
go through the same journey of self-discovery,
it's what makes life magical and meaningful.
If you think a hero is too strong a word,
wait to see your life unfold...
it'll be nothing short of heroic.
Take your time, you got this.

Carmen Oliveira

Connect The Thoughts!
Jot down notes and self-reminders here.

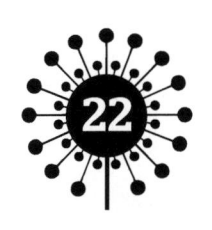

FOMO VS JOMO

Are you missing out for the right reasons?

**Power is not
given to you -
you have to take it.**

BEYONCÉ

FOMO VS JOMO

Are you missing out for the right reasons?

Years ago, I signed up for a school trip. There were at least 60 kids on this adventure and I was really looking forward to the experience.

Where I was going is irrelevant. Especially when you're 16. It's all about who you are going with, and who you will sit next to on the bus.

Months before our departure, we had a few meetings where our group of 60 were divided into two groups of 30 and we could ask the staff anything we needed to know about our trip.

I was placed in a group where the kids were speaking a language that I wasn't used to. It was the English language, but it wasn't the way I spoke, or behaved. It wasn't wrong, it was just different and unfamiliar. The staff that was assigned to our group, was an older version of these kids. I sat in my seat, looking and feeling like a lost deer in a forest.

"It doesn't feel right," said my gut.

The next group of 30 kids were sitting in a circle and talking and behaving like me. I wanted to get up and go sit with those people.

After staring at the other group for too long, my head turned back to my group and my forehead crinkled from thought. Was I put in my group for a reason? Should I stay and stick it out? Maybe the experience of being with these people will be good for me. The whole situation wasn't sitting right.

I needed to make a change.

I went home. Spoke to some friends and my parents. I thought about what it would be like to be with the first group, which was nervous, scared and not myself and what it would be like to be with the second group, relaxed, and totally myself. I decided to make my move. I switched trips.

Trip day arrived. As I got settled into my seat on the bus with the group that I switched to, I could see the other group through the bus window. I actually felt like I won something. Really big. I was so happy that I listened to my intuition.

Years later, when acronyms such as FOMO (Fear of Missing Out) and JOMO (Joy of Missing Out) became popular, my mind went right to this story.

If I had stayed with my original group, I would have probably hid in my hotel room while having complete JOMO and FOMO from not being on the group I switched to.

The best part? I found one of my best friends on that trip and I can't imagine life without her.

THE MORAL OF THE STORY:

Every day you are given the opportunity to make a choice. It could be as small as what to have for a snack to as big as if you should spend the summer volunteering in Cambodia. Listen to your gut to make your decision. It's your power and your move.

Ritual: Trust Your Gut

When you question whether you can trust something or not, that is when you already know that you can't.

Do you know that in order to survive and thrive you must trust your gut? How many times in your life have you said "I knew I shouldn't have done that"?

The five basic senses are, Touch (skin), sight (eyes), hearing (ears), smell (nose), and taste (tongue). Your gut instinct is often called your sixth sense and it is so important that it often overrides your choices even when the other five senses influence your decisions. Remember that no matter how good something looks, if it doesn't "feel" right than you should probably walk away.

Making good decisions, paying attention to your "inner voice", and knowing even without really knowing why may help to save you from harm, and other unpleasant day to day situations. You know those butterflies that you sometimes experience in your tummy? You know that feeling of regret that you experience when you realize that you ignored your gut feelings? These are the messages that you need to listen to even when they're telling you something that you really don't want to hear.

Listening to your gut is a feeling and thinking skill that is ever evolving and know that you have just as many "brain" cells in your gut as you do in your head. So the next time you are faced with a difficult situation, purposely ask yourself "how does this feel?" ... and don't look for the answer you want, instead accept the "true" answer those feelings give you. And finally, remember your gut isn't always tuned into your "happiness". It can give you messages that disturb, surprise, anger, and confuse you. You might like to revisit The Three Brain Meditation in Chapter 8 now!

The Trust Your Gut, or Rotated Wide Lunge, is a movement pattern designed to stimulate your gut. Exercises with built in core or gut rotations not only wake up your gut, but they also have the power to stimulate and build that all important connection between your head brain and your gut brain.

Practice: Trust Your Gut

ROTATED WIDE LUNGE

How to do the Rotated Wide Lunge:

Start in a comfortable standing position.

Bend forward and place your hands on the floor about shoulder width apart.

Step your feet back into high plank.

From high plank lunge your right foot up beside your right hand.

Raise your right hand straight up and rotate your upper body into right leg.

Put your right hand back onto the floor.

Step your right foot back into high plank.

Repeat the same sequence using your left foot and left hand.

Don't do this:

Don't forget to breathe.

Don't rotate from the raised arm and shoulder.

Don't compromise your spine.

Do this:

Make sure you rotate from your mid-body.

Keep your shoulders strong.

Lunge the foot right up beside the hand so that the lunge is big.

THE BOTTOM LINE:

Your brain can play tricks, your heart can be faint,
but your gut is always right!

Mentor Memos

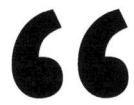

> Follow that feeling in your heart.
> Notoriety and accolades are great,
> but they won't define true happiness.
> Be fearless - not everyone will
> identify with your success,
> but they will all identify
> with your struggles.
> Be honest and share.
> It will impact people far and wide,
> without even realizing it.
> Be nicer to your siblings,
> they're your best friends.

Jordan Wagman

> Be happy and comfortable
> with who you are first
> and the rest will follow.

Agathi Yap

Connect The Thoughts!
Jot down notes and self-reminders here.

Get (Para) Sympathetic

Controlling your nervous system.

> Between stimulus and response
> there is a space.
> In that space is our power
> to choose our response.
> In our response lies our
> growth and our freedom.
>
> VICTOR E. FRANKL

Get (Para) Sympathetic

Controlling your nervous system

"You do realize that the other cars are driving way faster than you." My son informed me the other day in the car.

"Yeah, and?"

"Don't you care?

"Didn't even notice."

Why is there a need to drive fast and pass other cars? There was no hurry and we weren't late, I thought to myself.

Back in the caveman and dinosaur days, danger was everywhere. We didn't know where our next meal was coming from, or if we were going to be someone's next meal either. We have inherited from natural selection, the fight or flight reaction in our nervous system to protect us and help us flee from danger in a moment's notice.

Face to face with a bear? Standing on the street and a car is driving right at you? Your sympathetic nervous system has got you covered. Watch how fast you are able to get out of danger.

Getting back to the car ride with my son, the back seat driver. If I were to put my foot on the gas and zoom and swerve in and out of lanes at lightning speed to where I was going, sure, I would get there fast.

I don't feel the need to say "Outta my way" with my car and put my life and others in danger. In addition, there will be no medal waiting for me. Nor a pot of gold or even a gold star sticker for getting to our destination that way thanks to my parasympathetic nervous system, that is calming and sweetly whispering to me, "You will get there when you will get there".

Adults driving aggressively can explain a lot, but how do you know if a child has an unbalanced nervous system?

When they yell at the top of their lungs when someone doesn't put back the marker in the right case.

Huge red flag.

Act like this for a while and you may end up feeling completely drained and filled with anxiety over things that you shouldn't feel anxiety about.

THE MORAL OF THE STORY:

Overusing the sympathetic response will increase everyday stress. Reserving this "fight or flight" response for real danger will help with your long term mental wellness.

Ritual: Is Your Window Open

Controlling your response to the things that happen to you in life is a skill that can be learned and made better.

Did you know that you have the power to choose how you respond to every situation that you are faced with?

Your brain is essentially the boss of your body, but it can't do the job all by itself. Your nervous system connects the messages from your brain to your body so you can do things like feel, breathe, think, laugh, cry, and walk and talk. It is your information super highway and it controls everything you do by constantly responding and adapting to all the things that happen to you everyday.

Your ability to control your feelings is called self-regulation or being inside your "window of tolerance", and it is something that can be understood, practised, and strengthened ... these skills can be acquired and expanded upon at any time during your life. The best way to achieve this is by taking a moment between how something or someone makes you feel and how you respond to those feelings. Taking the time to think, work through your emotions, and then reacting to the situation shows that you are connected and tuned into not only yourself but the situation as well.

Healthy self-regulation is also about spending time outside your comfort zone in unregulated states. We learn so much about ourselves when we are hyper-aroused or in "extreme sympathetic" (the times when we just can't calm down), or are hypo-aroused or in "extreme parasympathetic" (the times when you are unmotivated and non-present). Spending time outside your "window" can offer you the opportunity to more fully understand yourself and your feelings.

Alternate nostril breathing, is a simple breathing technique that helps to calm your frazzled mind, body, and emotions. It can have a direct impact on your nervous system and it is particularly helpful for relaxing racing emotions, improving your ability to focus, and releasing anxiety and stress. "Breath control" exercises can help you manage difficult situations and also help if you are having trouble falling asleep. They are amazing tools to help balance, clear, and quiet your mind.

Practice: Is Your Window Open?

ALTERNATE NOSTRIL BREATHING

How to do Alternate Nostril Breathing:

Find a comfortable position either standing, sitting, or lying down.

Bring your right hand to your face and put your index and middle finger on your face between your eyebrows, lightly using them as an anchor. Your right thumb and ring finger will be used in the practice. Close your eyes and take a relaxing breath in and out through your nose.

Close your right nostril with your right thumb and
inhale through your left nostril.

Close your left nostril with your ring finger so that
both nostrils are closed and hold the inhale briefly.

Remove your thumb, open your right nostril and
release your breath slowly through the right side.

Pause briefly at the bottom of the exhale. Inhale slowly through the right nostril. Briefly hold both nostrils closed again at the top of the inhale.

Open your left nostril and release your breath slowly through the left side.

This is one complete cycle. Repeat 5-10 cycles, following your inhales and exhales.

Don't do this:

Don't breathe too quickly or too deeply.

Don't stress if you mix up the breath cycle, just pause,
centre yourself, and begin again.

Don't count if the numbers throw your focus off ... just breathe.

Do this:

Make sure your breath is slow and steady.

Be consistent with the length and hold of each your breath cycles.

Stay connected to the movement of breath into and out of your body.

THE BOTTOM LINE:

Alternate nostril breathing is a great way to press
the "reset" button the next time you need to find balance.

Mentor Memos

> Be honest.
> Be reliable.
> Be kind.
>
> *Tracy Brightmore*

> Slow down and enjoy the ride. Get out of the way and let things flow.
>
> *Cody McElrea*

> The best advice I have ever received is from my 99-year-old mother: "Don't worry too much; relax; calm down; take it easy. And, if the sky collapses, think of it as a cover/blanket over your body."
>
> *Susan Mok*

> Do your best at being your you-est you. Everyone is just trying to do their best. Including your parents!
>
> *Frances Policarpio*

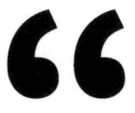

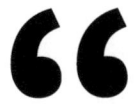

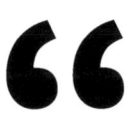

Connect The Thoughts!
Jot down notes and self-reminders here.

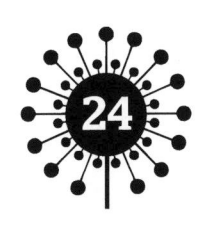

Getting Rooted

*Fast foot facts and
why you should care about
where and how you stand.*

**Stand straight,
walk proud,
have a little faith.**

GARTH BROOKS

Getting Rooted

*Fast foot facts and why you should
care about where and how you stand.*

When I was in middle school, there was a girl named Jill who carried a lot of power. People seemed to gravitate toward her. She was smart, yet quiet. Some called her pretty. In my eyes, she was more striking. Almost magnetic. She wasn't directly mean, although her friends were. The one thing about Jill that I found to be quite fascinating was that she was friends with Sandy, a girl who was on the opposite end of the social ladder.

Jill allowed Sandy to "stand" with her crowd. At recess, I would find Jill surrounded by her friend group while Sandy stood on the outside. Sandy stood a little taller than usual when she hung around Jill and her crowd. She would look around and smile, too.

When Sandy was with Jill and her friends, nobody would ever dream of telling her to leave. When not hanging around Jill and her crowd, Sandy had her own friend group, and was quite content with them.

At such a young age, Jill was able to be friends with whomever she wished. An obvious act that should be attainable, but unfortunately only a few can accomplish. It was so kind and generous that she gave some of her power to another and in doing so, Sandy obtained stability to stand tall and proud on her own two feet.

The story could be the same 30 years later, but with "likes" or with group selfies with those we admire.

It may seem shallow and ridiculous to feel proud just because you are "standing" with certain people; nevertheless, it is a necessity and meaningful for others who need a little push to feel grounded. Especially in middle school.

Where you stand and who you stand with says a lot about who you are and how you feel. There is no shame in reaching out to a powerful source for help, but after a while, you just may want to step back and realize that you probably had the power to stand all on your own.

THE MORAL OF THE STORY:

Getting a little help from your peers can give you the confidence you need. Knowing how and when to reach out for help can be an asset to your success.

Ritual: Feet On The Ground

When you are grounded you feel centred, confident, less tense, and less stressed.

Did you know that your day-to-day worries are best managed by a strong connection to the earth?

We all deal with worry at some point in our lives. Worry is a normal response to stress and it often prepares and motivates us to deal with overwhelming situations. Think about the times in your life when you had to give a speech, study for a final exam, prepare yourself for a competition, or go out on a date with someone you were interested in. These are all situations that could cause you to feel apprehension, worry, and a sense of being ungrounded.

A few things you need to remember about worry are, that it has absolutely nothing to do with strength or courage. It happens when your brain perceives danger even when there is no danger, and that literally everyone experiences worry as a common occurrence at some point in their lives. Worry builds strength, it challenges you to be courageous ... remember, without worry there would be no need to be brave.

The best way to overcome worry is to learn how to ground yourself. The feeling of being "grounded" is usually described as feeling "rooted" to the earth and one of the best ways to do this is to kick off your shoes and walk barefoot in the grass. You know that the sun provides you with warmth, energy, and vitamin D. Did you also know that the earth is a source of grounding energy as well?

Your feet are your first level of ground contact so they are very important in the process of grounding. It is really important that you take good care of them and that they are strong and healthy. The well being of your feet is a major contributor to the well being of the rest of your body. Foot rolling is a great way to care for your feet. Rolling gets rid of aches and pains, stimulates blood flow, and releases tension. Foot rolling also wakes up and stimulates your foot muscles after they've been tucked into a pair of shoes for *hours.*

Practice: Feet On The Ground

FOOT ROLLING

How to Foot Roll:

Find a comfortable standing or sitting position.

Place a small ball (about the size of a golf ball) under the instep of your foot.

Lean against the ball with a little bit of your body weight.

Roll the ball around the entire sole of your foot.

Do the same thing with the other foot.

Don't do this:

Don't put too much weight on the ball.

Don't avoid the tender spots, just apply less pressure.

Don't forget to breathe.

Do this:

Spend as much time in your bare feet as possible.

Make sure you roll your toes as well.

Roll from your heel right through your instep (right up and into your toes).

THE BOTTOM LINE:

Happy feet ... happy body. Stand tall, grounded, and proud!

Mentor Memos

"

You're allowed to like a variety of music.
No matter what other kids may tell you.
Explore a variety of sports. Not a fast runner?
Who cares! You are still an athlete!
You're living in a Golden Age of
music and pop culture: Appreciate all artists.
Always wear the Docs with a dress. :)

Sandra Pozzobon

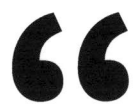

"

Not everyone is going
to understand you,
and that's okay, as long as you
take the time to understand yourself.

Yashar Khosroshahi

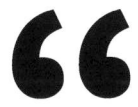

"

Don't over think it - just get out into nature,
in hindsight you will always be grateful for it.

Fern Hoffer

Connect The Thoughts!
Jot down notes and self-reminders here.

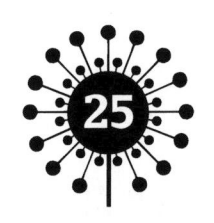

Change the Scenery

Choose what you want to look at wisely.

Sometimes all you need is a change of scenery.

JAY KASLO

Change The Scenery

Choose what you want to look at wisely.

The Baby Bjorn is a baby carrier. This device allowed me to carry my infant son like a kangaroo. In a pouch that was fastened to my upper torso.

We began to use it the moment he was born and it was very convenient and useful. I could do many things when he was in my "pouch." My hands were free so I was able to make a meal and talk on the phone at the same time. Productive.

I liked to place my son facing me, so it would feel like I was hugging him and he would feel warm and secure.

One day, when my son was 3 months old, I decided to go for a walk. I put him in the Baby Bjorn, just like I always did, facing me. This time he wouldn't stop crying.

I tried taking him out and putting him back in. I even added a stuffed toy. Nothing. He kept wailing every time I put him in the device. The amusing thing was that he stopped crying when I took him out to try again.

My gut instinct told me to face him outwards.

He stopped crying and began to make happy baby sounds.

He wanted to see.

Although he was only 3 months old, his developmental progression awakened his sensors which lead to his desire to see where we were going and what we were doing. The original direction, facing me, was no longer good for him because it blocked his view.

What would happen if we took this mentality of my three month old son and brought it into our daily lives? To listen to our gut instinct and decide what is good and not good for us to see and experience.

Wait until you feel the freedom and satisfaction that my son felt. Although my son couldn't speak at the time, it was obvious.

THE MORAL OF THE STORY:

Don't like what you are seeing? Change the view. Instant satisfaction.

Ritual: Around The World

One of the best most nurturing and healing environments is "nature".

Did you know that your surroundings have a direct impact on your mood?

Everyday, all day, you are affected by your surroundings ... both in good and not so good ways. There is always something good to be derived from where you are, even if it's a little tiny thing like recognizing that your whereabouts are not positive, not nurturing for you, and need to change. Understanding this leads to solutions, which leads to change, and change leads to positive outcomes ... as soon as Sharon (as she described in this chapter) understood that her baby wanted her to change the way he was being carried, the crying stopped and he became happy.

One of your biggest life struggles is that your surroundings are not always under your control and this lack of control often causes you to experience fear and anxiety. Creating healthy surroundings can play a huge role in supporting and helping you feel comfortable and balanced and they can also have a very strong effect on your mental, physical, and emotional well being.

Another important thing to consider is that your "happy place" might be someone else's "unhappy place" ... also a place that once made you comfortable might shift and no longer provide the same source of happy inspiration. Moving forward, pay attention to how your surroundings make you and others feel, and if they are not working for you, change them so that they do!

The Around the World Jumping Jack is the perfect exercise to give you a constantly changing view. The jumping jack is an invigorating and easy cardio move that involves both upper and lower body movement. It can be done with impact to drive up the intensity or done in a low impact version to make it less stressful. The around the world version of the jumping jack has you adding quarter turns to your jacks so that you are facing another direction. If you do this four times you will have gone "around the world".

Practice: Around The World

TRAVELLING JUMPING JACKS

How to do Travelling Jumping Jacks:

Stand up straight with your arms by your sides and your feet about hip width apart.

Jump to a wider stance and at the same time raise your arms out to the side and over your head.

Jump again and return to your starting position.

This is one jumping jack.

Now, do eight jacks, then a quarter turn.
Then, eight jacks, then a quarter turn.
Then, eight jacks, then a quarter turn.
Then, eight jacks, then a quarter turn.
Then, reverse your direction until you are back at your starting point, taking you "around the world".

Don't do this:

Don't flail your arms.

Don't jump too high or too wide.

Don't forget to breathe.

Do this:

Make sure you bend your knees to absorb the shock
on the landing of the jump.

Keep your body in a strong upright position.

Change the number of jacks in each direction - instead of eight, try four, or two ... it will change the intensity!

THE BOTTOM LINE:

Changing your environment can make
a huge difference - and it is easy to do.

Mentor Memos

"

Do what rocks your soul.
Take chances, try hard things, fall down, stumble, get up, sing at the top of your lungs, play loud music, spend as much time in nature as possible, and be kind to yourself.
Nothing comes to stay, it comes to pass, and you will be a different person when it does - tomorrow, in a week, a month .... that includes obstacles, friends, insecurity, acne ...

Make stuff. Anything. With food, with dirt, with clay, with pen and paper, with your community. Just keep putting stuff together and see what you can create.
Feed yourself good food, clean air, lots of water, plenty of laughter, abundant hugs, lots of sleep ... what you put in your body matters and influences how you feel, how you think, how you move, how you relate to yourself, to others, to your environment, to life.

Terry Walters

Connect The Thoughts!
Jot down notes and self-reminders here.

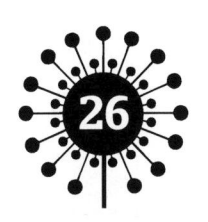

Centred Strength

It's amazing what can throw you off balance.

**I've never been
one to sit back and go,
"I'd better do what the
audience wants me to do, because
I don't want to lose them".**

JIM CARREY

Centred Strength

It's amazing what can throw you off balance.

When I was in my early 20's, I worked as a counsellor on a bike trip for a teen travel camp. I was actually a camper with the same company when I was 15, so I thought it would be neat if I had the chance to give back what my counsellors gave me when I went on the same trip.

Role models.

Friendship.

Feeling safe.

That did not happen. At all.

My campers did not reciprocate to my warmth, mentorship, and friendship.

I wish I could say that with a little time and patience, my campers came around and we all got along so well that on the last day, we couldn't release each other from our hugs, and tears were streaming down our faces because we didn't want our trip to end.

Once again, that did not happen. At all.

I remember arriving home and standing in my apartment elevator thinking that I am not meant to have kids. I can't do it. It's too hard. I'm not the type because I obviously failed at the simple task of being a counsellor.

After a while, I began to reflect and look at the whole picture.

This wasn't my first time at this rodeo.

I was a counsellor several times before and it was a positive experience on both sides.

I took a hard look at my campers from this challenging trip. I realized that most of them had personal issues that weighed heavily on them and as a result, they were all unappreciative, disrespectful and downright mean.

I should have never thought that I failed. If anything, they failed me. They missed out on me.

Being a counsellor on this bike trip knocked me out of my core. During the trip, I noticed that I lost my balance and dropped like a rag doll from the abuse. Time passed. My strength returned. Even though I really never lost it. It just seemed that way.

THE MORAL OF THE STORY:

Observing the whole picture and all of the moving parts that go with it allows you to see where you went wrong, or didn't. Even though that summer was a difficult one, I didn't quit. I stuck it out and finished a difficult task that taught me that sometimes no matter what you do, your audience may not accept you, and that's ok. There will be others.

Ritual: Gut Punch

Any and all muscle that sits above your mid-thigh and below your floating ribs is your core ... 360 degrees! And yes your butt is included in your core!

Did you know that your breath and body power are intimately connected?

It is important to remember that the primary purpose of your body is to move ... to get you from here to there in a balanced, efficient, and powerful way. Think of the engine of a car and how it is essential to moving the car ... your core is your body's engine and its strength affects the strength of your whole body which in turn influences your physical and mental health and wellness.

Your connection to your breath and its effect on your body power is what moving well in your body is all about. Think about a professional tennis player and how they grunt at the very same time they're hitting the ball back to their opponent. The timing of this grunt and its purpose are not only crucial to them hitting the ball with maximum power but also the accuracy of that power. The forced exhale in the form of a grunt and its perfect timing with the movement results in a dramatic increase in physical prowess and power.

So let's take this one step further and talk about how connecting to your breath and core not only makes you stronger but also takes you closer to achieving your goals! Your breath and centre (core) affect your emotions, your emotions affect your mental game, and your mental game leads you to a greater and more balanced life that is filled with achievements, stability, and success.

The Gut Punch Crunch is the perfect exercise to help you establish a strong connection to how natural it is to breathe or exhale when you are contracting your core muscles. In fact, the muscles that are involved actually have the dual function of making both breath and power happen. Once you learn about this natural and magical connection you will realize that you do this many times during your day. For instance, when you lift something heavy, when you get up from a sitting position, and when you exercise.

Practice: Gut Punch

GUT PUNCH CRUNCH

How to Crunch:

Lie flat on your back in a comfortable position.

Poke/press your fingers into the sides of your abdomen and contract it as if you are being punched in your gut.

Another way to activate these muscles is to cough which is a forced exhalation.

Now try to activate the same muscles on your own without the "gut punch" or cough (see below).

Don't do this:

Don't hold your breath.

Don't make the contraction too violent.

Don't forget to think about the contraction.

Do this:

Try raising your shoulders up off the floor at the same time as the cough or forced exhale.

Slow the forced exhale down for a longer and deeper "gut" contraction.

Make sure you understand how to contract these muscles without the forced exhale ... at will.

THE BOTTOM LINE:

If you want to move well, look well, and feel well you have to move from your core!

Mentor Memos

"

No matter what it looks like,
everyone has insecurities,
we all want to be loved,
and we are all created equal.
We are all born perfect beings full of love,
and it is your mission to follow
the bliss that lies within your heart.
Shine your unique light into the world,
and be an example of the kind of love
that you would like to receive.
The universe will take care of the rest,
and provide opportunities
for you to learn and grow.

Carrie Neiss

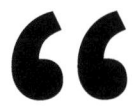

"

No matter what situation you are in,
always, always trust your gut instinct.

Lidia Wojcik

Connect The Thoughts!
Jot down notes and self-reminders here.

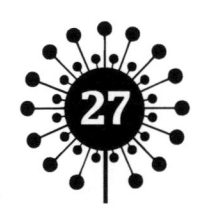

Motivation and Discipline

*They seem the same,
but they're so different!*

All successes begin with self-discipline. It starts with you.

DWAYNE "THE ROCK" JOHNSON

Motivation and Discipline

They seem the same, but they're so different!

"Yup, it's Adhesive Capsulitis. Otherwise known as Frozen Shoulder."

Said the physiotherapist.

I had pain in my shoulders for months. I tried to ignore it, but after I couldn't raise my hands to wash my hair any longer, I knew I had to do something about it.

"And?" I asked.

"Well, you can come here for a few sessions, but you need to do several exercises on your own to help it heal properly."

I made a sour face. I'm all for exercise, but only exciting and fun exercise. You know, spinning classes, tennis, running. Things that get my heart racing and my body sweating.

I received 5 exercises to do with a ball and a stretchy elastic thingy. They were easy, slightly painful and exceptionally boring. When was I going to do them? I thought. And do I really need to do them?

Although I didn't say these words out loud, it was as if the physiotherapist heard me.

"You need to do them. Or it will get worse."

I nodded. I felt as if I got a D- on a test.

I had my homework cut out for me.

I put the exercise instruction sheet and equipment on a chair, in the corner of my bedroom and left them there. The next day, I went to a spinning class.

For the next couple of days, the exercise instruction sheet moved. As I walked passed it, I created a slight breeze that was strong enough for it to gently lift up and land on my bedroom floor. I left it there.

A week later, in the shower, I knew I couldn't raise my hands to wash my hair, but now I couldn't raise my hands to wash my shoulders. It was getting worse. I had no choice but to begin the exercises ASAP.

I was not motivated to do the exercises because they weren't fun and exhilarating, like my spinning classes were. I began to realize that motivation is led with your heart and it's attached to emotions. Discipline leads with your head. No matter what you feel, you do what needs to be done. I knew I had to heal my shoulders and I needed to be disciplined to do it.

Motivation did not have a role here. It was almost as if it took a back seat. And so I began. And I began again. And again until it became a routine. Although it was not easy, I tried to make it as pleasant as possible. During the exercises, I watched TV and I listened to music.

Two weeks later, I returned to the physiotherapist and I could raise my arms to reach my shoulders. I made progress, but I had a lot more to do.

Good thing I had discipline.

THE MORAL OF THE STORY:

If you want something, regardless of your motivation, you need to do whatever it takes to get to that goal. The more you have discipline and grit, the more goals you can accomplish in life.

Ritual: The Motivator

The origin of self-discipline and motivation was originally your "survival" (think caveman). Today this is no longer the case.

Did you know that self-discipline and motivation are two very different things but actually work hand in hand?

Discipline is about changing your behaviour so that you are in control of any given situation. Imagine that really boring history exam that you have to study for. The only way you're going to learn the course content and pass the exam is by sitting down into a chair and forcing yourself to read and learn ... there really is no other way. At the root of self-discipline and motivation is "understanding", and here in lies the disconnect. If you understand, I mean when you REALLY understand that a situation needs to change than you change it ... it's that simple. It's when you reach the point of understanding "need" that motivation is sparked and you create change ... otherwise nothing happens. As Sharon shared in this chapter, even though she knew the consequences of not doing her physio, she didn't really "get it" until the pain and loss of movement got worse! The light bulb went on, she really understood, and she was motivated to make the change!

Self-discipline and motivation work off of each other. Motivation can be fostered and created from self-discipline ... when you commit to being disciplined enough to get something done, and when your motivation waivers, self-discipline can take over and keep you going until you get the job done. Most importantly they both lead to feelings of accomplishment, pride, and feeling good!

The Motivator is a high and low intensity exercise. It is the perfect combination of strength building and cardio conditioning. Using your own body weight will make you stronger - and because The Motivator involves so many big body movements and level changes, it will have a positive impact on making your heart and lungs stronger.

Practice: The Motivator

THE ALTERNATIVE BURPEE

How to do The Alternative Burpee:

Stand in a comfortable position with your feet about hip width apart.

Raise your hands above your head and jump straight up.

When you land back on your feet, squat down and place hands on the floor.

Hop or step your feet out behind you so that you are in a high plank position.

Hop or step your feet back up to your hands.

In one big motion bring yourself back to an upright position and hop.

This is one burpee.

Don't do this:

Don't rush through them.

Don't let your back arch during the plank.

Don't land too hard.

Do this:

Make sure you breathe.

Modify the movements if you are tired or not strong enough to do them yet.

Pause during plank and make sure your core muscles are fully engaged.

THE BOTTOM LINE:

Where there's a will, there's a way.

Mentor Memos

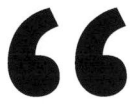

> People make choices, choices have consequences.

Lisa Damour

> Always travel with open eyes and an open mind. Seek advice when you need it and never turn down unsolicited advice. Never say never because it just may end up being part of your career or life journey. This advice is coming to you from a surgeon-scientist who started out thinking they would be a music teacher, then a scientist and never dreamed of being a doctor let alone a surgeon. Life is full of surprises!

Mary Nagai

Connect The Thoughts!
Jot down notes and self-reminders here.

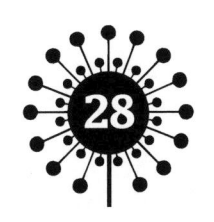

21 Days to Form a Habit

*Before you know it,
it will be like second nature.
It just takes a little practice.*

**The truth is,
you don't break a bad habit;
you replace it with a good one.**

DENIS WAITLEY

21 Days to Form A Habit

*Before you know it, it will be like second nature.
It just takes a little practice.*

"I know my keys are somewhere…" My friend and roommate Deena kept saying, over and over again as she looked feverishly through every pocket of every pair of pants, jacket, sweatshirt and purse.

"Arrgghhh." She groaned as she paced up and down our hallway.

I plunked down in our beanbag chair and waited. I reapplied my lipstick.

"Ah! Got them! - They were in my red purse."

"Let's go!" I said as I stood up.

We had a movie to catch and I really didn't want to miss the previews.

On the subway, I had to say it.

"You know, there's a way to stop this from happening again."

"From what happening again?" Deena innocently asked.

She obviously forgot about her missing keys.

"Your keys. There's a way to prevent misplacing your keys!"

"Like when does this ever happen?" She asked with a giggle.

"ALWAYS!" I yelled back.

Deena smiled.

"They need a home. A special place just for your keys so you will always know where they are, every time. No questions asked."

"Yeah - I know where my keys are." Deena said with an annoying tone.

"Sure you do." I said sarcastically. "You know what? Just try it — as an experiment — for fun."

"Ok - but it won't work." Deena said.

And for the next three weeks - 21 days, Deena placed her keys on a hook just above the light in her room.

It wasn't easy. I had to remind her a few times to make sure she put her keys there.

On day 22, I asked "Where are your keys?"

"Okay!" Deena laughed.

Being organized grants you freedom from distractions.

THE MORAL OF THE STORY:

Although it's difficult at first, each day you practice your new healthy habit, you will get closer and closer to allowing yourself to focus on your main goals.

Ritual: 21 Day Push-Up Challenge

A habit is usually a consistent and involuntary behaviour that you perform daily.

Did you know that your life is essentially the sum of all of your habits, both good and bad?

Your life is shaped by your rituals and habits. They determine how happy or unhappy you are, how successful or unsuccessful you are, how physically fit you are ... and maybe even how to set yourself up so that you always know where your keys are! So it would be safe to say that you are the sum of all of the little habits and decisions you make during your day-to-day life.

Yes! Habits are routines that we perform daily, and they can be physical, mental, and emotional. Also, think about the "Domino Effect" of your habits. Think about the weight you could gain or lose by changing your eating habits, or the time you could save or waste by knowing where your keys or phone are. Think about the positive emotional impact that could come from small changes and how this could ultimately lead to your mental health and wellness.

Ideally, you want to develop good habits, ones that lead you to feeling good about yourself and the best way to do this is by making conscious and positive decisions. This means that positive habits can lead you to become the best version of yourself rather than causing a negative impact on you in the long run. Good habits can lead to dramatic life improvements.

Whether you perform an amazing push-up or not, the 21 day push-up challenge is guaranteed to make you stronger. A really good push-up is one of the most powerful exercises that you can do with just your own body weight. This exercise can strengthen your core, triceps, biceps, shoulders, back, glutes, and more. In addition to helping build strength, the push-up can also build mental and emotional resilience!

Practice: 21 Day Push-Up Challenge

THE PUSH-UP

How to do a Push-Up:

Drop down onto your hands and knees.

Place your hands on the floor a little wider than your shoulders.

Straighten your legs and come up onto your toes into a high plank position.

Bend your elbows and let your chest and body drop down toward the ground.

Your elbows should bend out and away from your body.

Drop down to a 90 degree bend at your elbow and stop.

Push yourself back up into a soft elbow (don't lock out your elbows at the top).

This is one push-up.

On day one do one push-up, Day two do two, Day three do three and so on until you reach 21 push-ups on day 21!

Don't do this:

Don't let your lower back sag.

Don't forget to breathe.

Don't lead with your head and neck.

Do this:

Keep your shoulders and neck relaxed.

Place your hands a little wider than your shoulders.

Make sure you fully engage your core muscles.

THE BOTTOM LINE:
You are the sum total of your habits!

Mentor Memos

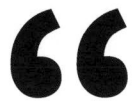

"

No one should ever be allowed to compromise
your integrity, so cut out the "people-pleasing".
You have the power to bring your ideas to life,
so pack the criticism of others who
don't share your core values
in your ignore box.

Joy Badler

"

Attune to your voice,
values, and uniqueness.
Know that love isn't based
on someone else's opinion
of your "correctness" but
that it is unconditionally yours
to receive from within.
For when we love ourselves more,
we fortify our "original medicine".
The world needs more of that.

Melissa Leithwood

Connect The Thoughts!
Jot down notes and self-reminders here.

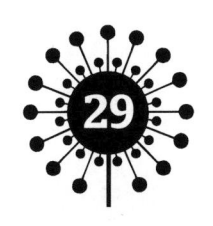

From BFF to SFF

The Changing of a Friendship.

**Make new friends,
but keep the old;
Those are silver,
the others gold.**

JOSEPH PARRY

From BFF to SFF

The Changing of a Friendship.

Elaine and Patricia met at camp in the summer of 1968 and they were inseparable. They were BFF (Best Friends Forever). At the time Elaine was living in New York and Patricia was living in Chicago so after the summer they kept in touch throughout the school year.

Obviously, there was no email or social media back then and long-distance phone calls were expensive.

They wrote (by hand!) long letters to one another. Once a year Elaine took the train to see Patrica and vice versa.

The following year, Elaine went overseas to university. That meant no visits or phone calls for a whole year and Patricia was heartbroken! They had to write only letters and WAIT a LONG time to get them.

During the late '60s and early '70s, Elaine and Patricia were in each other's lives - a lot.

When Patricia was in her mid-twenties, a job opportunity came up in New York, where she met her husband and had two children.

As the years passed, Elaine and Patricia started to become friends with other people. Their kids went to different schools. Life got busy and they both began to realize that their friendship was changing.

The time in their lives when they were close was for a reason.

Their lives became different. They were different.

What did they do about it?

Nothing.

They became SFF - Special Friends Forever.

Now both in their seventies, they meet to play cards every Wednesday. They love to talk about their life together and just the other day, Elaine said to Patricia "We always find our way back to "Us".

THE MORAL OF THE STORY:

Enjoy the friends you have now. They are in your life for a reason. Accepting the fact that friends come and go in your life can help you to handle change, which is a guarantee in life.

Ritual: The Side Bend

Much like the flexibility that trees blowing in the wind have, you can become very good at adapting to changes in your friendships ... both new and old.

Did you know that one of your most basic needs in life is the presence of other kind humans? Did you also know that one of your body's most basic needs is for it to be strong and capable of moving in all directions?

If you think about it, you likely get from where you are to where you want to go in a straight line - that makes it quick and efficient, which is great! BUT, it's important to move in many directions/dimensions. Why? It's great practice for when you need to deal with difficult situations ...when things go sideways! When you learn and practice moving in all dimensions, you will be able to do everything better in life (really!).

For example, moving your body sideways helps you build power, skill, flexibility, and adaptability. The side bend is a perfect way to do this. When you bend your spine sideways, it causes your muscles on one side to shorten and at the same time causes your muscles on the other side of your body to lengthen. This give and take is an essential skill - for your physical body and so much more. It will help you move sideways better and we all know that being able to give and take is important in every way to have and hold good friends.

Imagine that as you practice the side bend, you are building skills and creating a "friendship" in your body ... this will have short term and long term benefits in the same way that having a good friend will.

Practice: The Side Bend

CONTRACT AND RELEASE

How to do The Side Bend:

Stand in a comfortable position with your feet slightly wider than your shoulders.

Bend to the left side and slide your left hand down the outside of your left leg.

At the same time slide your right hand up the right side of your rib cage toward the underside of your shoulder.

Return to the starting position.

Bend to the right side and slide your right hand down the outside of your right leg.

At the same time slide your left hand up the left side of your rib cage toward the underside of your shoulder.

Repeat the motion on both sides 10 to 12 times.

Don't do this:

Don't make your range of motion too big.

Avoid jerky movements.

Do this:

Keep your neck and hands relaxed.

Keep your movements smooth.

Use your breathing to assist the side contractions.

Make sure you keep your core muscles engaged to support your lower back.

You can try adding light weights once you understand the move if you want this exercise to help you build core power.

THE BOTTOM LINE:

Your body needs to be able to give and take at the same time ... it will prepare you for everything life (and friends!) brings your way.

Mentor Memos

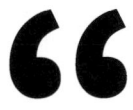

"

Careful what you post online,
it will outlive you.

Joanna Salit

"

You have a purpose in life.
A reason for being here.
Look around for it...
you'll find clues everywhere.
Listen to what people say
you're good at and build
on those good things.
Collect experiences and build
your purpose organically as it
grows, adjusts, and clarifies.

Nancy Kopman

"

Nothing is permanent -
this too shall pass.

Kailey Gilchrist

Connect The Thoughts!
Jot down notes and self-reminders here.

Catch Your Breath

*When it all becomes
too much,
take the time to
just breathe.*

**Never be ashamed
of what you feel.
You have the right
to feel any emotion
that you want, and to do
what makes you happy.**

That's my motto.

DEMI LOVATO

Catch Your Breath

When it all becomes too much, take the time to just breathe.

From the moment I saw her open the car door, it was all over her face. "Bad day!" My daughter declared. "I tried to get extra help in chemistry and there were too many students and not enough teachers. Lisa is not talking to me and Neil is completely avoiding me for no reason. Nobody likes me, I hate school. It's too hard." I quickly caught on that there were too many things on her plate. It was "too much".

"What about Biology? You like Biology, especially Ms. Lee." I gently suggested.

"Meh - whatever."

I could feel the weight of her angst and frustration and she was doing a great job throwing it all on me. Psychologist Dr. Lisa Damour explains in her book *Untangled*, "Teenagers often manage their feelings by dumping the uncomfortable ones on their parents." A book not to be missed for validation for living and understanding the ups and down of a teenager.

I let her continue and decided to drop her off at home while I made a quick grocery run. Secretly I wanted to give her time to cool off.

Take time to get it out.

When I got home, I presented her with one of her favourite snacks. Then I let her let it all out. She ranted. Yelled. Screamed. Questioned. I listened as I stroked her hair. When she did say something that was, in my opinion, silly such as quitting sciences just because she is having trouble on one assignment, I said something like "Do you think the

Wright Brothers got to fly on the first try? Science is hard. It's ok to struggle. Its part of the growth."

You need to stop. Breathe. And do something that calms you.

"Can I take a bath?" She asked between tears.

And off she went.

Later that evening, I met her in the kitchen. As she opened the fridge for a nighttime snack, "You ok?", I asked. "Yeah - I get it now. It just took a while."

I smiled as I took a deep breath and hoped my daughter did the same.

Life can be overwhelming. Take the time to let it out and breathe and then do something that you enjoy.

THE MORAL OF THE STORY:

Learning how to deal with stress far exceeds what you gain by taking academic subjects. Life comes with wrong turns and bumps in the road and you need to acquire the skills to manage through it.

Ritual: HIIT

HIIT stands for High Intensity Interval Training. It's a fast and challenging workout that has a really good effect on your mind, body, soul, and also your ability to deal with everyday stresses.

Did you know that HIIT training is a great way to teach your body how to deal with different kinds of physical and mental stress?

It is also an amazing way to get a quick fix and to change up your workouts so that you don't get bored. When you learn to push yourself to be breathless and then recover and catch it again, you are building coping skills for life ... resilience, strength, and confidence.

Tabata is a fun and challenging kind of HIIT workout. This fast paced challenge is made up of short intense bursts of energy followed by either active recovery like walking, or brief periods of complete rest. There is nothing boring about Tabata, and the best thing is that you will be finished before you even know it. The whole workout takes four minutes!

Tabata can help you reach your goals of becoming stronger, leaner, faster, and it can also give you endurance.

Another powerful thing about Tabata is that it builds power in your head, heart, and lungs. This workout is good for any level of fitness from beginner to intermediate to elite athletes. You can use this HIIT workout for just about any exercise including jumping jacks, push-ups, sit-ups, squats, swimming, cycling, running, skipping rope, etc.

Enjoy catching your breath!

Practice: HIIT

TABATA

How to do Tabata:

One Tabata workout consists of 8 x 20 second intervals with 10 seconds recovery (total workout time is 4 minutes per exercise).

Choose an exercise! Full body exercises to get a harder workout (push-ups, jumping jacks, burpees etc.) or simple exercises to build strength in specific areas of your body (lunges, pull-ups, planks etc.).

Workout hard (80-100% capacity) for 20 seconds.

Rest for 10 seconds.

This is one interval.

Repeat the same interval eight times.

Beginners can start with four or five intervals. Intermediate and advanced participants can do the whole four minute workout.

Don't do this:

Don't do this workout more than one or two times weekly.

Don't let the quality of your movements change when you get tired.

Don't push yourself to the point of injury.

Do this:

Warm your body up before you start the workout.

Start with four or five intervals if this is a new workout for you.

Rest for 60 seconds between sets of Tabata.

THE BOTTOM LINE:
You need to be able to handle any challenges that land on your plate ...
exercising is a great way to develop coping skills ...
when you practice, you will be able to catch your breath.

Mentor Memos

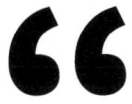

> Do not overthink what others think.
> *Jaime Slavin*

> If it doesn't feel right, it probably isn't right, for you.
> *Ellen Schwartz*

> You need the sad things to happen so that you can heal from them and become stronger. There is a purpose to the harder emotions in life. They teach you how to heal yourself and find a better connection to your truest self. What seems like a lot of struggle and challenging times, will actually become your superpower! You never know who you will inspire, just by being you and braving your way forward!
> *Nastasia Irons*

> Value your body, you've only got one … it's the foundation that you will have for the rest of your life.
> *Lynda Thomson*

Connect The Thoughts!
Jot down notes and self-reminders here.

The GET UP Glossary

words to live by

Accountable: The act of making sure you do the thing you said you would do.

Act of God: An event that is out of your control, but is in the control of a higher power.

A Hit: A serving of a recreational drug.

Adhesive Capsulitis: When you can't move your shoulder due to stiffness. Immobility takes place in the shoulder joint. Should not be ignored and must be treated with the proper medical attention.

Angst: A feeling of deep anxiety or dread. One who feels this, requires some serious attention, like a hug.

Aunt Flo: A term to describe menstruation.

Auto Pilot: The act of going through daily tasks or rituals without any emotion.

Avoiding: Staying away from a person or object.

Awakening: A sudden realization.

Awesomer: A notch up from awesome.

Ass-Power: The physical act of sitting down on your gluteus maximus (ass) and working for an extended period of time.

Balance: Feeling emotionally and physically stable.

Bearable: Something that can be tolerated.

BFF: Acronym for Best Friend Forever. A term to describe a treasured friendship between two people.

Bottom Line: The most important thing to be considered.

Brave: Executing without fear getting in the way.

Breath: Taking air in and letting it out. Helps calm anxiety, support energy and exercise. Essential to our health and well-being.

Breathe: The practice of Breath. A requirement for all living things. A function that we need to be reminded about, especially during stressful situations.

Brew: Soaking, boiling and fermenting a product, but also can be described to prepare a task.

Challenging: A task that is difficult, but is welcomed to be accomplished.

Chaotic: Unorganized and out of control.

Change: An occurrence that makes something different and is inevitable.

Chef: Master of a recipe.

Chisel: The act of cutting away at an object or subject in order to get to an end goal.

Chirped: To speak to someone in a teasing or taunting way.

Chore Du Jour: Non-negotiable things to do that need to get done each day.

Cleaning: The act of making something clean, free of dirt and anything you want to rid yourself of.

Comfort Zone: The space where one feels comfortable. No growth or learning is accomplished.

Confidence: The feeling of being certain about someone, something and most importantly, yourself.

Confrontation: When two people who are on opposing ends, communicate.

Core Muscles: The area of muscles in the middle region of your body.

Counteract: To work against something in a way that encourages it to be right.

Counterintuitive: The opposite of what makes sense, but actually ends up working.

Cruel: Another word for mean.

Curious: A feeling that you want to learn more. Promotes great learning and growth.

Decadent: Appearing to be self-indulgent, rich, and of a luxurious nature.

Deflated: A feeling of being emptied of energy.

Destination: The end to your journey, and perhaps a great accomplishment.

Detours: A guide to go another way.

Discipline: A way to behave and work by following a set of rules.

Disease: When something in one's body goes wrong.

Distractions: Things or people that get in the way of what you are doing.

Domino Effect: When an action causes a series of effects or events.

Doormat: A place to wipe your feet - something you don't want to be mistaken for.

Dopamine: The "feel good" hormone that helps us thrive and focus.

Drained: A feeling of fatigue or lack of energy.

Dumping: Objects or feelings that are considered waste and disposing it/them.

Elated: Extreme joy or happiness.

Emotion: A description of feelings that should be acknowledged and never ignored.

Energy: A feeling of strength and vigour in order to accomplish physical or mental activity.

Estrogen: Hormones that promote the development and maintenance of the female body.

Euphoric: An incredible wave of happiness.

Exhale: The act of letting out a breath. Should be accompanied by inhaling and done frequently.

Experiment: The act of testing something to obtain a result.

Extraordinary: An ordinary thing or moment that grows to a different level.

F.A.I.L: Acronym for First Attempt In Learning.

Failure: An act that doesn't execute.

FOMO: Acronym for Fear Of Missing Out.

Freedom: The ability to act without restraints.

Friendship: A platonic and supportive relationship between two people.

Friend Group: A collection of friends that you spend time with.

Frustrated: Distress or annoyance ... can cause your body to feel tight.

Ginormous: A blend of giant and enormous. Extremely large.

Grateful: Appreciating something or someone.

Gratitude: Showing appreciation.

Gravitate: To be attracted to someone or something.

Greens: A highly nutrient dense green food, most likely a vegetable or fruit.

Grind Your Gears: Describing something or someone that gets on your nerves.

Grit: Using as much perseverance, courage and determination to achieve a goal.

Grounded: Being able to stand in a healthy emotional and physical state.

Growth: When someone or something increases. Usually occurs after a struggle.

Guck: A slimy, dirty, or unpleasant substance.

Gut Instincts: A decision that you feel within your soul.

Habit: A subconscious ritual.

Happy: Feeling of elation that should be strived to achieve as much as possible.

Happy Place: Somewhere where one feels elated.

Hardwired: Automatically thinking or behaving in a particular way.

Healthy Habit: A ritual that benefits your well being.

Hippy Dippy Freaky Flower Child: Someone light and fluffy.

Home: Place of residence for a person or object.

Homework: Work that needs to be done outside of supervised instruction. Requires discipline.

Hot Potato: A situation that is difficult to deal with, causing a lot of stress ... makes you want to drop it, like a hot potato.

Humiliating: Extremely embarrassed to the point that you want to stick your head into the ground.

Hunched Over: When your head and shoulders slouch forward, creating a hill in between your shoulders and the back of your head.

Insecurities: Having a loss of self-worth. The opposite of secure.

Inseparable: When two people or things are unable to be apart.

Instinct: A knowing or natural understanding or impulse

Intuition: The ability to understand and direct action without any outside help. Best achieved through your gut or a higher power.

JOMO: Acronym for Joy Of Missing Out.

Journey: Travel time to your destination, which can be filled with incredible growth.

Kicker: An unexpected or unwelcome turn of events.

Kinesiophere: The Akira Concept's term for the fluid-state energy you are enveloped in. It is controllable, receptive, broadcasted, and shared.

Kindness: The act of doing something kind. Do this as often as possible.

Kyphosis: See Hunched Over.

Language: Method of communication. When understood by more than one person, expression of thoughts can be exchanged.

Logical: Orderly, consistent, and reasonable.

Me Time: Time carved out, to do anything, especially for you.

Meh: A neutral reaction that does not contain any excitement.

Melancholy: Sadness.

Mentor-like: A person who offers worthy advice and direction.

Mistreat: The opposite of how you want to be treated.

Molly: MDMA. A psychoactive drug used for recreational purposes, also known as ecstasy.

Monthly Cycle: A term to describe when a woman is menstruating. See Aunt Flo.

Motivation: To obtain a reason for behaving or acting a certain way.;

Mood: A conscious state of mind or emotion.

Narcissistic: Someone who feels they are better than anyone else.

Nervous System: A collection of nerves that sends messages from the brain to different parts of the body.

Notable Alumni: Memorable people who attended an institution of some kind.

Off Balance: Feeling physically or emotionally not stable.

Overwhelming: When an activity or person becomes too much to handle.

Pandemic: The worldwide spread of a new disease.

Parasympathetic Nervous System: Slows your heart rate and calms you down during a situation that requires attention.

Perfect: Having all of the required elements as best as they can be.

Perseverance: Never giving up, despite a challenge.

Persistence: Continuing with something even though it is difficult.

Perspective: How you see things. Great opportunity to change.

Poop: Bowel movement, obtained by a healthy diet.

Power: Complete control of a situation

Practice: Accomplishing an activity over and over again to perfect it.

Premenstrual Syndrome: Any combination of emotional, physical or psychological disturbance that occurs after ovulation.

Prep Day: Taking the time to prepare what you need for what is ahead.

Priorities: Crucial things that need to get done.

Progesterone: A hormone that stimulates the uterus to prepare for pregnancy.

Process: A series of steps to accomplish before a task is completed.

Putter: To travel between destinations.

Reciprocate: Giving back what you just received.

Reflect: Taking the time to think about what occurred.

Rejection: Denying entry or acceptance, which probably is a blessing in disguise.

Reinvent: Thinking up a whole new way of doing something.

Resilience: The act of recovering quickly after a challenge, perhaps slightly stronger than before.

Response: An answer.

Rep: An abbreviation for a repetitive act when exercising.

Roadblocks: Things that get in the way of your end goal. Nothing to be afraid of. Walk around it, jump over it, or whip it up in a blender.

Routine: A series of rituals to be done daily.

Sanity: The psychological state of your well being.

Screaming Match: A competition of screams. Who can be the loudest?

Second Nature: Doing something with great ease, due to practice.

SFF: Special Friend Forever. A description of a meaningful friendship between two people.

Smoothie: A thick smooth drink made from pureed raw fruits, vegetables, and a liquid.

Snug As A Bug: A feeling of coziness. Ideal feeling during relaxation time.

Stand: The act of obtaining an upright position. The question is, how upright can you be?

Stimulus: Some sort of activity or energy in response to something.

Stir The Pot: To deliberately change a situation to cause a reaction.

Stress: The result of emotional and/or physical pressure.

Squat: The ideal exercise for the Gluteus Maximus. Otherwise known as the butt.

Step Up To The Plate: Ready to work on the job at hand.

Struggle: Working through a challenge with some degree of force. Not a comfortable situation. May promote growth.

Subconscious: Part of your mind that you are not fully aware of, which influences all actions.

Success: An act or project that occurs with a favourable outcome.

Supine: Lying down with your face upwards.

Sympathetic Nervous System: Places you in "Fight or Flight" mode. Helps your body react in dangerous situations.

Tenacity: A determination to continue what you are doing with persistence.

This: An object or situation that is pointed out with thought.

Timing: A point or period of time, when something happens.

Uncomfortable: The opposite of comfort, where growth can bloom.

Us: A term for two or more people who carry a bond.

Veggie: Shortened version for vegetable. A nutritious food source.

View: What you are able to see right in front of you. Completely changeable, if required.

Visualization: The formation of a mental visual image.

Wait: What you need to do in between starting something and ending it. Will require much patience.

Weight-Bearing Exercise: Physical exercise that challenges your muscles, enabling them to get stronger.

Wisdom: Acquiring knowledge through life experience.

Whirlwind: When air moves around a lot. Can be described as a feeling of too much activity going on.

Whoa: A command to stop whatever you are doing, immediately.

Worthwhile: Something that is worth your time.

Zigzag: Alternating your movements from side to side, left and right.

zzzz: Sleep.

GET UP Mentors
get to know them

CHAPTER 1

Marci Warhaft
Author of The Good Stripper: A Soccer Mom's Memoir of Lies, Loss and Lap dances. One of Canada's top 100 health influencers.

David W. Eisen, MD, CCFP, FCFP
Physician

Gordie Arbess, MD, CCFP
Physician, HIV/AIDS Primary Care Specialist, Cycling Enthusiast, Experienced Dad.

CHAPTER 2

Linda Kessler Shapiro
Sales and Marketing Professional, Newly Minted Ceramicist, Proud Mama.

Wendy Chong
Executive Presentation Skills Coach

Megan Khosroshahi
Director of Execution and Evolution at Borden Communications and The Akira Concept.

CHAPTER 3

Leslie Josel
Author of How to Do it Now, ADHD Academic Coach, Owner of Order Out of Chaos, Creator of Academic Planner: A Tool for Time Management®

Christopher Wong
Urban Farmer

Sandy Kruse
Holistic Nutritionist

CHAPTER 4

Nicholas Ferguson
Co-Founder, TheGreatUnited.org

CHAPTER 5

Leanne Matlow
CBT Counsellor and Workshop Facilitator, Author, SPACE (Supportive Parenting for Anxious Childhood Emotion) Provider, Creator of Mental Health Empowerment Day MHED.

Melanie Levcovich
Consultant for Alternative Investments and Family Philanthropy. Business Advisor, Project Give Back.

Betsy McLeod
IT Professional, Morning Walker and Fitness Enthusiast, Introvert Extraordinaire.

CHAPTER 6

Debbie Berlin
Psychotherapist

Ryan Storm
We Move Through Stormy Weather Podcast, Public Speaker, Accidental Activist.

CHAPTER 7

Debra Basch
Lifestyle Coach

Hope Paterson
Entrepreneur Coach. Travel, Food and Innovative Education Specialist.

CHAPTER 8

Martin Perelmuter
CEO of Speakers Spotlight

Peter Neal
CEO of Neal Brothers Foods, Mental Health Survivor, Advocate, Food Lover.

CHAPTER 9

Navaz Habib
Chiropractor, Author of Activate Your Vagus Nerve.

Stacey Jackson
Singer/Songwriter and Television Presenter.

Naomi Strasser
PR Executive, Reformed Teenager.

Krystyna Roberts
Truth Seeker and Mother of two awesome humans.

CHAPTER 10

Nancy Ramadan
Nature Enthusiast, Lover of Life, Grandma.

Liz Waisberg
Social Worker and Outdoor Enthusiast.

IJ Schecter
Bestselling Author

CHAPTER 11

Dawn Lane
Teacher

Jody Shulgan
Active Citizen who really cares about kids

Karen Gnat
Yoga/mindfullness/nutritionist who specializes in trauma awareness for youth and adults

CHAPTER 12

Lisa Kates
Photographer and Building Roots Partner.

Kev Self
Curious Idealist, Human Designer, and Coach.

Lisa Borden
Unconventional Idealist, Innovator, Instigator and Initiator. Producer, Get Up.

Andrea Scher
Author and Artist.

CHAPTER 13

Rich Knox
Drummer and Good Human.

Kathleen Sommerville
Well-being Enthusiast

CHAPTER 14

Govind Kilambi
Investment Professional

Shannon Coleclough
Culinary Mushroom Farmer, Farmers' Market Champion, Mother of 2

CHAPTER 15

Oren Epstein
CEO Bio Raw

Richard Carmichael
Father (of hens & humans), baker, builder, writer, business wrangler. Owner, Grounded Pantry.

CHAPTER 16

Brian Phillips
CEO of WORLDSalon and WORLDHairSkin.

Ryan Golt
Mental Health Advocate

CHAPTER 17

Colleen Kavanagh
Founder of ZEGO LLC

Rob Storm
Active Dad, Sales Guy, Musician.

Lisa Binns
STUSH Executive Chef and Chief Artisan.

CHAPTER 18

Judy Librach
Host of Finding Your Bliss on Zoomer Radio, Life Coach, Author, and Speaker.

Maria Biber
Senior Interior Designer

CHAPTER 19

John Mason
Learning Activist at Sideways

Noa Daniel
Teacher, Consultant, Author, TEDx and Keynote Speaker.

Dayna Freedman MD FRCSC
Obstetrician and Gynecologist, Peleton Enthusiast, Proud Mother of two.

CHAPTER 20

Marla Gold
Movement/Wellness Educator. Event Planner and Project Manager. Innovator.

CHAPTER 21

Carmen Oliveira
Educator

CHAPTER 22

Agathi Yap
CEO of Harmonized Fitness and Wellness

Jordan Wagman
James Beard Nominated Chef, Author, Culinary Cannabis, Philanthropist, Host, 'In The Weeds' Podcast

CHAPTER 23

Cody McElrea
Plant Medicine Distributor. Natural Medicine Worker.

Susan Mok
Active Citizen

Tracy Brightmore
Portrait Photographer

Frances Policarpio
Soul Seeker, unapologetically resistant to anything "should".

CHAPTER 24

Sandra Pozzobon
Educator

Yashar Khosroshahi
Brain Based Executive Coach and Co-founder of MINDSHIFT LEADERSHIP.

Fern Hoffer
Active Citizen, Nature Lover, Proud Mama of 3.

CHAPTER 25

Terry Walters
Clean Food Chef, Author, Educator and Adventurer - in the kitchen and in life.

CHAPTER 26

Carrie Neiss
Artist

Lidia Wojcik
Reiki Practitioner and Dreamer.

CHAPTER 27

Lisa Damour
Psychologist. Mom. Author of NYT bestsellers UNDER PRESSURE & UNTANGLED.

Mary Nagai
Surgeon-Scientist

CHAPTER 28

Melissa Leithwood
Mama, Wellness Advocate, and Giver. Advocate for mental health and liberated expression.

Joy Badler
Educator and Life-long Learner.

CHAPTER 29

Nancy Kopman
Early Childhood Educator, Composer/Performer.

Kailey Gilchrist
CEO and "Sauce Boss" at NONA Vegan Foods Ltd.

Joanna Salit
Hard to define, but ... Social Worker, Therapist, and Parent of 3.

CHAPTER 30

Jaime Slavin
Registered Dietician and Masters Public Health.

Nastasia Irons
Naturopathic Doctor, Spin Instructor, Runner, Creator of @salt.water.wellness

Ellen Schwartz
Founder of Project Give Back, Author of Lessons from Jacob, and Without One Word Spoken.

Lynda Thomson
Spiritual Advisor

ACKNOWLEDGEMENTS

I was always planning on writing a second book, but I had no idea that it would be a book like this.

I am grateful and thankful for the following people.

LISA BORDEN, these three words you said to me in your office changed my life. "Yes, you can." I looked at you like you were crazy, but you ignored me (that was a good thing) and held out your hand and I didn't let go. I am in awe of your expertise, attention to detail, and tenacious spirit to care for our world.

My partner in crime, DAVID NEWTON. A man who nearly threw me out of his spinning class many years ago for my annoying flip phone that wouldn't stop beeping. Little did we know what was in store for us years later. Collaboration, support, and teamwork like I've never seen before. David, you have taken the art of moving your body to a whole new level of wow.

ROB STORM, your colourful commentary makes me smile each time I enter the Borden Communications office. JOANNA SUGAR, could I have a more wonderful and meticulous neighbour? Thank you two for your excellence and thoroughness in editing.

Where would I be without MEGAN KHOSROSHAHI? Your patience, digital expertise, and kind gentle manner make any daunting task that has to get done doable.

To each and every thoughtful and generous MENTOR. This book would not be complete without your wisdom. Thank you for sharing your meaningful answer to the burning question that everyone needs to know: "What would you tell your teenage self?" I know that your words will have an incredible impact on someone's life.

JOSH, ADAM, and LIV ARBESS. Parenting at its finest! You guys have taught me more than I would have ever imagined, and provided me with great content to share - and I didn't even ask your permission! Please don't kill me. Love you, my sweeties!

GORDIE ARBESS, the world needs to know that this is what happens when you support me when I fall down, cheer me on when I succeed, and leave me the heck alone when I'm writing. There is no one I'd rather be riding this rollercoaster life than you. I love you more than you know.

Last but not least, I wouldn't be here, still standing, without my FRIENDS, you know who you all are. To my PARENTS and sister CARRIE. We've all come a long way since Cressy Rd. I'm proud of it. I thank you and love you for building my foundation.

THE COVER STORY

Why imperfect grass and a dandelion?

We want you to be you ... authentic and perfectly imperfect ... just like the grass. Dare to grow in your own way. Don't compare yourself to others, the grass is greener where you water it.

None of us are the perfect shade of green, manicured to perfection - appearance is superficial and isn't what matters. And a weed? That's just a label. The dandelion belongs - it grew there for a reason and is beautiful and resilient!

Your life, like your lawn is all yours - tend to it, care for it, enjoy it, and accept it for it's uniqueness and how it grows!

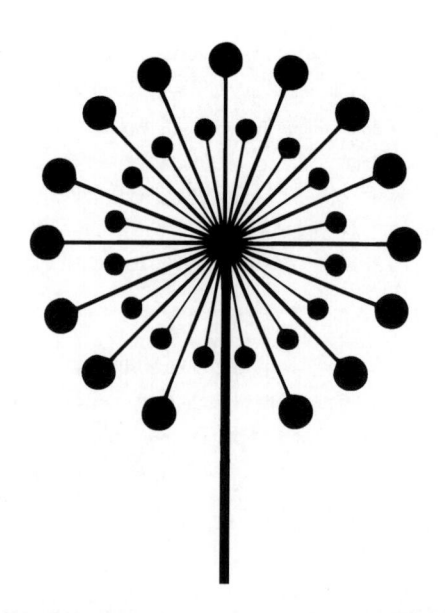

Manufactured by Amazon.ca
Bolton, ON